The Green Smoothie Prescription

ALSO BY VICTORIA BOUTENKO

Raw Family: A True Story of Awakening

*12 Steps to Raw Foods: How to End
Your Dependency on Cooked Food*

Green for Life

*Green Smoothie Revolution:
The Radical Leap Towards Natural Health*

*Raw Family Signature Dishes:
A Step-By-Step Guide to Essential Live-Food Recipes*

Raw and Beyond (co-authored with Chad Sarno, Elaina Love)

CHILDREN'S BOOKS:

Green Smoothie Magic

I Love Greens

A Gift from Little Bear

Fruits I Love

The GREEN SMOOTHIE PRESCRIPTION

A Complete Guide to Total Health

Victoria Boutenko

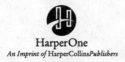

HarperOne
An Imprint of HarperCollinsPublishers

HarperOne

This book contains advice and information relating to health care. It should be used to supplement rather than replace the advice of your doctor and other trained health professionals. If you know or suspect that you have a health problem, it is recommended that you seek your physician's advice before embarking on any medical program or treatment. All efforts have been made to assure the accuracy of the information contained in this book as of the date of publication. The publisher and the author disclaim liability for any medical outcomes that may occur as a result of applying the methods suggested in this book.

FIRST HARPERCOLLINS PAPERBACK EDITION PUBLISHED IN 2016

Designed by Terry McGrath
Illustration by Katya Korobkina

ISBN 978–0–06–233654–5

Library of Congress Cataloging-in-Publication Data
Boutenko, Victoria.
The green smoothie prescription : a complete guide to total health / Victoria Boutenko.
— First edition.
    pages cm
ISBN 978–0–06–233652–1 (hardcover)
1. Nutrition. 2. Smoothies (Beverages). 3. Fruit juices. 4. Vegetable juices. 5. Functional foods. 6. Health. I. Title.
RA784.B63886 2014
613.2—dc23   2014022239

16 17 18 19 20 RRD(H) 10 9 8 7 6 5 4 3 2 1

To all those who dare to take a stand for their own health.

Contents

Dear reader,

Do you eat enough greens? If you don't know, I have more questions for you. Do you hiccup regularly? Do you sigh a lot? Do you have painful knots in your back? Is your vision blurry? Do you have lots of wrinkles? Do you crave chocolate all the time? If you answer yes to any of these seemingly unimportant questions, you're probably not eating enough greens.

Dark leafy greens contain an astonishing abundance of nutrients that are vital to good health. However, since the beginning of the industrial revolution two hundred years ago, the diet of people in the Western world has undergone a dramatic change: they almost completely stopped consuming fresh greens, along with the proper amount of fresh fruits and other vegetables, and added lots of refined and canned products. Processed foods, as we know now, not only lack important nutrients, but also contain preservatives and many other chemicals harmful to our health.

As a result, people started acquiring countless nutrient deficiencies, which increased from generation to generation, inevitably causing serious health problems. Certain groups of people who sustained themselves mostly on processed and refined products developed such severe diseases as scurvy, rickets, beriberi, and pellagra. Today we know that pellagra is caused by a chronic lack of niacin (vitamin B3), and scurvy is a result of vitamin C deficiency and can be cured by simply eating limes. However, by the end of the nineteenth century these ailments continued to take many thousands of human lives year after year. For example, in 1915, more than 10,000 people died of pellagra in the United States alone.[1]

As we continue to consume a lot of processed foods, the deterioration of our health continues today. Astonishingly, 133 million Americans—almost 1 out of every 2 adults—have at least one chronic illness.[2] Seventy percent of Americans take prescription drugs[3] and more than 35 percent of the American people are obese.[4] Based on available statistics, the number of totally healthy people in America seems to be rather small—despite the fact that the United States spends over $3 trillion a year on health care.[5]

Every human being, just like every other creature on the planet, has the right to health. This is our natural state. And yet something is amiss; we're not as healthy as we deserve to be. So how do we return our health to its natural state? Could it be leafy green vegetables?

During the last two decades, there has been a noticeable increase in the amount of global research on the health benefits of greens. American nutritionists now recommend three to five servings of greens daily. This might sound like a lot at first, and I understand why some might think it's difficult to consume a healthy amount of greens per day, especially if you're trying to do it through salads alone. Children, in particular, don't want to eat salads, and adults get bored eating the same thing at every meal. That's why I believe green smoothies are the perfect solution to lasting good health.

Green smoothies are the easiest, fastest, and most delicious way to consume the amount of greens necessary to sustain a healthy and fun lifestyle.

In August 2004, I created the first green smoothie in my office in Ashland, Oregon. Inspired by many positive comments, I wrote an article titled "Ode to Green Smoothie" and e-mailed it to everyone in my Internet address book. Almost instantly people responded with raving feedback and detailed testimonials. The number of people who were drinking green smoothies turned into a "green smoothie tsunami," which continued to grow throughout the summer.

After that I dedicated a year to thoroughly researching all of the nutritional data available at that time about green smoothies. In October 2005, I published *Green for Life*, which was literally the only book about green smoothies available until Robyn Openshaw published her *Green Smoothies Diet* in 2009, nearly four years later. Since then, many other authors have published books about the power of green smoothies.

At first, I was happy about the popularity of green smoothies, as it was my dream to spread the news about this healthy drink to the entire planet. However, I soon discovered that some authors recommended adding sugar, dairy, chocolate, salt, coffee, oils, supplements, and even alcohol to green smoothies, the very ingredients green smoothies are designed to neutralize. As a result, people didn't feel better after consuming green smoothies and published their opinions online, which started to drown out the very real and scientifically sound good news about green smoothies. Rather than helping to spread this good news, many of these new books only confused the issue.

This twist in the course of events disappointed me personally, because I have put a huge amount of time and energy into this research and I strongly believe that if green smoothies are consumed properly, they are nothing but beneficial. By popularizing this healthy drink, we can enable millions of people in the world to significantly improve their health.

Between 2008 and 2013, I conducted nineteen green-smoothie retreats, at which participants consumed only green smoothies for seven days. The outstanding healing effect of green smoothies on more than a thousand participants confirmed the scientific research about the vital role of greens in the human diet. I believe that increasing the daily consumption of fresh greens can help many people restore their health naturally to the way it was when they were years younger, which is why I decided to write *The Green Smoothie Prescription,* an essential primer for great health that includes all of the best available scientific data about the benefits of green vegetables. But it's not just science. There are also delicious recipes, inspiring success stories, and personal anecdotes about my life living on greens.

I hope this book will inspire you to include green smoothies in your daily meals. With this, I raise a cup of green smoothie to your health!

—*Victoria*

1 What We Learn in Childhood

The greatest obstacle to discovery is not ignorance—
it is the illusion of knowledge. —DANIEL J. BOORSTIN

Most of our habits and beliefs about food are shaped in early childhood. In my research I came upon studies about childhood imprinting. Flavors in a mother's milk, I was amazed to learn, shape a baby's later food preferences.[1] What's more, during weaning—what psychologists call the "sensitive" or "critical" period—a child starts to store specific powerful thoughts and associations about food based on what the child eats as well as watching what other people eat, especially the mother. This imprint, according to psychologists, is almost irreversible; later events have little or no effect on a child's preference for food.[2]

That is why different nationalities have different food preferences. People in Asia, for example, eat a lot of rice. Latin Americans swear by corn, Russians adore bread, Italians enjoy spaghetti, and so on. Food choices are even more diverse when it comes to appetizers. One group feasts on caviar and raw fish. Another savors oysters, snails, or countless other rarities. It is interesting that each group might find another group's "delicacies" disgusting. Still, we continue to cling to our distinctive food choices as if they were the only way to eat. It happens because our food preferences are ingrained in us, literally.

When I was young, my father worked as a pharmacist. At home, in a small chest, among gauze pads, bandages, and cotton balls, he kept two main medicines with which he treated all of our family's health problems. I recall that my father gave us aspirin if we had a fever, which happened approximately once a year, and another bitter-tasting pill if we had a sore throat or any other pain. I remember that those treatments occurred routinely, and I never questioned their validity and was certain that all people did the same. I appreciated their convenience but wondered how these medical drugs worked. My father, even being a pharmacist, could not explain to me how a tiny pill placed into a mouth could control the pain in a completely different part of the body.

As part of his profession, my father studied medicinal herbs and taught my little brother and me about the restorative powers of pine needles, nettles, dandelions, sorrel, golden root, chaga mushrooms, and various other medicinal plants.

We lived on the Russian island of Sakhalin, near Japan, and our winters were long, cold, and snowy. Beginning in February, our bodies lacked vitamins, so my father showed my brother and me how to collect the young pine needles and chew a small bunch of them regularly. In May, when the first dandelions sprang from the ground, I helped my father pick their leaves, which we mixed with sauerkraut and oil as a salad. Then, in the summer, we regularly picked stinging nettles and cooked a nettle-potato soup. Almost every Sunday my father and I went to the forest and brought back baskets of wild berries. Unfortunately, the addition of wild edibles to our food didn't seem significant to me at that time; rather, they were fun and saved our family money. Only decades later, as I look back now, do I recognize how precious this education was and that it laid the foundation for my genuine quest for natural healing.

When I was sixteen, I graduated from high school and took a nine-hour flight to Moscow, where I entered State Pedagogical University. I wanted to be an art and English language teacher and a nurse. At that time, in the Soviet Union, all female university students who were studying to become teachers were required to become medical nurses. We went to school six days a week. One day a week was dedicated to studying medicine. Our lectures were conducted not only in classrooms, but also in hospitals and even the morgue.

I enjoyed and admired the medical profession with all my heart—until I went to work as a nurse at a local children's hospital. That's when my rosy dreams of being a "good fairy in a white robe" were crushed by the solid reality of sickness. I remember watching children suffer all kinds of discomfort. The pediatricians and nurses there performed various procedures, but all their manipulations didn't seem to help much. I felt helpless and disturbed. After just a month, I quit my job. That was when I first started to question the limits of allopathic medicine and seriously started wondering about alternative remedies that could help those poor children.

However, I still believed that allopathic medicine provided the most progressive healing techniques. I continued to take aspirin whenever I had a fever, visited doctors if I felt sick, and meticulously followed all of their recommendations. When I got married and had my own child, I took my son to the hospital every time he got sick, which happened quite often. When the doctors prescribed loads of antibiotics and other pills, I was afraid to skip even one treatment because I was afraid that my son wouldn't get well. It didn't occur to me that there might be something the doctors didn't know.

For many years I thought it was unfair that some people would get ill and suffer, especially children. When my oldest son, Stephan, was five, he had his tonsils removed. I remember sitting helplessly at his bedside. My little boy was looking at me with those grown-up eyes on that pale little face, breathing heavily. I couldn't breathe I felt so much sadness watching my son's suffering.

Coincidentally, on the way home from the hospital, I met a friend and shared with her my sad story. To my shock she started yelling at me, accusing me of stupidity and cruelty. She lent me a book, Paul Bragg's *Miracle of Fasting*, telling me that I absolutely had to read it. I devoured it in one sitting. This book explained that poor health was not just hopelessly bad luck, but that our health, and the health of our loved ones, could often be greatly improved. Paul Bragg explained that the human body has the ability to heal itself if the proper conditions are provided, conditions such as good nutrition, clean water, fresh air, and others. His book opened my eyes to the fact that the human body is not our enemy but is indeed a friend, dedicated to our well-being. Instead of trying to treat the symptoms of illness, we could try removing the cause of disease, such as lack of nourishment, too many toxins, stress, etc. I was learning how I could improve my son's and my own health by following the simple advice of this author. For the first time, the general picture of human health was beginning to make sense to me. Even though my little son was still in the hospital, I was relieved by the thought that I would never make such a mistake again.

I was exactly one day late in reading Paul Bragg's book. Had it been only a day before, I would not have agreed to let my son undergo surgery. In desperation to share what I had learned, I started translating the book into Russian and copying it with a ballpoint pen on five layers of extra-thin paper with carbon paper in between. I spent all evening writing. It made me feel better. When my blue pen ran out of ink, I continued with a green pen, then a red one. I wrote through the night, finishing at daybreak.

I wanted to make a thousand copies and distribute them to everyone in Moscow, but there were no Xerox machines around at that time. I gave copies to a few close friends who, in my mind, needed a dose of Bragg's wisdom. Though I had put my own son through an unnecessary surgery, my friends would never have to subject their loved ones to such a procedure.

Perhaps I needed to go through a certain amount of pain before I could comprehend the simple truth about health: the human body has its own healing mechanism. It is programmed to repair itself naturally, without pills, ointments, or shots. Some complex physical injuries and severe illnesses and diseases require medical help, but the majority of our minor ailments, such as a headache, a sore throat, or a slight fever can—and should be—treated differently. In fact, a healthy diet and natural lifestyle often prevent such conditions. It was all so obvious to me. Right away, we, as a family, became vegetarians, bought a juicer, water-fasted on Mondays, and began swimming outdoors year-round. The effects were immediate, and for many years my family and I were strangers to disease.

How can I explain my feelings when I was reading the book? The impact this book had on me was radical and immediate, quite different, I'm sure, from its effect on the average American reader. Imagine a Russian woman reading a revolutionary book written by an American author. While reading it, I visualized a country where people regularly fasted on water and ate only healthy food. I dreamed of one day visiting and shopping at the Bragg Health Center in Los Angeles, which Bragg described so vividly in his book. Since the book had been published in 1966, I assumed every American had read it.

After reading *The Miracle of Fasting,* I started paying more attention to the food that appeared in American movies and magazines. I noticed that a lot of it was packaged individually in bright-colored paper, and all the ingredients, I heard through others, were listed on the package.

In the Soviet Union, on the other hand, most of the food was sold in bulk. I recall that in the 1970s I went to the store with several fabric bags that I sewed myself and purchased half a kilo of rice, a kilo of buckwheat, 200 grams of raisins, 200 grams of dry beans, and another kilo of potatoes, carrots, onions, and beets or other types of vegetables. If I didn't bring bags, the food would be packaged in paper bags, which would tear easily. To purchase oil everyone had a dark glass bottle. For milk we used a special enameled can. The milk was raw and unpasteurized, and it would become sour in two or three days. I only rarely found packaged foods in Moscow and other large cities. Somehow, I believed that Americans knew more about food than Russians, and that their food was "better for you." I also thought that the bright packaging with all the nutritional information on it was important. Enthusiastically, I kept sharing with my friends about health-food stores in America.

You can imagine my excitement, then, when in 1989 Colorado University offered me a position as a visiting professor of Russian Language and Art. Soon, my husband, my three children, and I arrived in Denver, ready to lead the life I'd always imagined in the United States.

Every convenience brings its own inconveniences along with it.
—LATIN PROVERB

Upon our first visit to the supermarket, I was delighted to find an abundance of bright, convenient packages. I was pleased to discover "low-fat" and "no-fat" foods, which we immediately loaded into our shopping cart, filling it completely. A smiling cashier invited us to use as many plastic bags as we wanted. Many times in my life I have observed how easy it is to form unhealthy habits, even when you know better. When everyone around you is falling for the ready-made convenience foods, you are more likely to do the same. And this is what happened to me and my family. Quickly and smoothly, hardly without a moment of protest, we adopted the American way of eating, surrendering completely to the Standard American Diet.

Staying busy with our life in the new country, we didn't notice how quickly we were gaining weight and how sick we were all becoming again. By 1993, my husband, our two younger children, and I became deathly sick. I was only thirty-eight, I weighed 280 pounds, and I was continuing to gain more weight. My legs were constantly swollen from edema. My left arm frequently became numb at night. I remember always feeling tired and depressed. I was diagnosed with arrhythmia, the same disease my father had at sixty-five.

At the same time, my husband, Igor, developed progressive hyperthyroidism and chronic rheumatoid arthritis, which made him feel perpetually fatigued. He was in constant pain and—to my horror—his doctor told him he'd have to spend the rest of his life in a wheelchair. I was afraid he and I would die, and our children would become orphans.

Our daughter, Valya, was born with asthma and allergies, but she never really had to worry about them in Russia. Her symptoms, at their worst, were mild. In Denver, however, she woke up almost every night with a cough that wouldn't stop until Igor gave her a lymphatic drainage massage. On top of all those troubles, our son Sergei was diagnosed with diabetes in September 1993. He was nine years old.

Of course, we discussed the possibility of adopting a vegetarian diet again, but it had somehow lost its appeal. Besides, we still didn't understand how poorly we were eating. We hadn't yet figured out the link between the Standard American Diet and our health. We thought we were eating healthy food, just like everyone else, even though not one of our American friends had ever heard of Paul Bragg or his book.

Mistakes are the portals of discovery.
—JAMES JOYCE

When I started searching for the cure for my family, my goal was to find a different solution, but one that would work for sure. I started reading medical books, but ended up back in the field of natural healing. I discovered raw food as a means to my family's health.

In January 1994, we became a "Raw Family." By turning off the pilot light in our stove and discontinuing all cooking, we were able to heal all of our life-threatening diseases. Even Sergei's blood sugar stabilized due to his new diet and regular jogging. Since beginning to eat raw food, he has never again experienced any form of diabetic symptoms. We were greatly surprised not only by how quickly our health was restored to normal, but by how much healthier we were than ever before. Our health improved so quickly, all four of us ran the BolderBOULDER 10K race within three and a half months.

Interestingly, my father and I suffered from arrhythmia simultaneously. Once I switched to a raw diet, my arrhythmia disappeared completely. My father, though, continued to follow his doctor's recommendations, taking pill after pill. He'd sometimes ask me to buy him some of the medications in the United States. I remember I felt so awkward driving to the drugstore and buying his pills. Soon my father suffered his first heart attack, and I invited him to come and live with my family. I was hoping to inspire him to include more fresh vegetables and fruits in his diet. My father lived with us for about a month, during which time he ate mostly raw food and went on daily long walks. When he left, he felt so much better, after just a month of eating raw food. Sadly, several years later, he suffered a second heart attack at the age of seventy-three. This one was fatal.

For the next seven years, everyone in my family lived on a raw-food diet. I stopped working at the university, and instead began organizing lectures and presenting on the raw food lifestyle. We began homeschooling our children and traveling extensively in the United States. During this time we gave many lectures and visited all fifty states teaching people about nutrition. During this time we published our first book, *Raw Family: A True Story of Awakening*. Eventually, we found ourselves living in Ashland, Oregon, where we started a business called Raw Family. And we felt fantastic. But as time passed, we each started to feel as if we'd reached a plateau. Our healing process seemed to have stopped. We started feeling discontent with our existing food program. I began to have a heavy feeling in my stomach after eating almost any kind of raw food, even a salad with a light dressing.

Finally, I narrowed my diet to fruits and nuts. I immediately put on weight. My family members felt confused about our diet and always seemed to ask, "What should we eat?" We were often hungry, but we didn't want to eat our typical raw foods: fruits, vegetables, nuts, seeds, and dried fruit. We felt trapped. I remember Igor looking inside the fridge, over and over again, and saying, "I wish I wanted some of this stuff."

At first, we blamed it all on overeating and were able to refresh our appetites with fasts, exercise, hikes, or working more. In my family, we strongly believed that raw food was the only way to go, and therefore we encouraged each other to maintain our raw diet no matter what. Many of my friends told me about similar experiences, at which point they gave up being 100 percent raw and began adding cooked food back into their meals. My family, though, continued with raw food due to our constant support of each other.

Meanwhile, we developed some small but noticeable symptoms of declining health, such as a wart on a hand or a gray hair, which brought doubts and questions about the completeness of the raw-food diet in its present form. Finally, we had to admit that we were missing something essential in our diet. When my children complained about the increased sensitivity of their teeth, I decided to conduct more research. I started collecting data about every single food that existed for humans. As my grandmother used to quote, "Seek and ye shall find."

After many wrong guesses, I finally found the correct answer. I found one particular food group that matched almost all human nutritional needs: greens. The truth was, in my family, we were not eating enough greens. Moreover, we did not like them. We knew that greens were important, but we never heard anywhere the exact quantity of greens we needed in our diet. We had only a vague recommendation to eat as much as possible. In order to find out the quantity of greens we needed to eat, I decided to see what animal research could tell me. The animal genetically closest to humans is the chimpanzee. Chimpanzees share an estimated 99.4 percent of their genes with humans. At the same time, these animals possess an extremely strong natural immunity to AIDS, hepatitis C, cancer, and other fatal human illnesses.[3]

When I realized the quantity of greens we humans are supposed to consume daily, which was approximately one pound, it became clear to me that I had to come up with an utterly new approach. From the study of human anatomy I learned that, for the best possible absorption, greens have to enter the digestive tract in liquid form. Greens are high in cellulose, which makes them difficult to break down. In perfectly healthy human bodies, in the absence of nutritional deficiencies, greens are broken down by two processes. The first is through chewing. The second occurs when the greens mix with the acid in the stomach.

At the time, I was already missing several of my molars, and my stomach acid was extremely low. Naturally, I started looking for a way to preliquefy large quantities of greens. At first I decided to blend dark leafy greens in a high-speed blender. Yet when I blended greens with water and opened the lid of my blender, the smell was unbearable. I quickly closed the lid and knew right away that I couldn't possibly drink that mixture. But I knew I was on the right track, so I continued to search for the best method.

Several days later, I came across a paragraph in Jane Goodall's book *The Chimpanzees of Gombe: Patterns of Behavior,* in which she mentioned that sometimes chimpanzees would take a fruit, roll it in a green leaf, and eat it as a sandwich. I stared at that paragraph in disbelief. According to human research, pairing greens with fruit is a poor food combination.[4] Then I thought to myself, "Maybe chimps know better."

I still had greens in my fridge. I also had bananas on the counter. I peeled the bananas and blended them with green kale. With trepidation I opened the lid of the blender. To my relief, it smelled sweet. I tasted the green drink, and it tasted exactly like a banana smoothie. I downed it. I consumed a large amount of greens without any resistance from my body or my taste buds. I didn't feel nauseous. To be perfectly honest, I enjoyed greens for the first time in my life! I started dancing right there in my office.

I decided to test my green concoction on other people. So I blended more kale with bananas, took a full pitcher of smoothie and some small paper cups and went outside onto the street near my office. There was a group of students there from the massage school next door. They were on their lunch break. I approached them and offered them my "very special treat." When these young people saw something green in my hands, they replied that they had just eaten lunch. I begged them to try it, and they reluctantly agreed.

As soon as they tasted it, their faces lit up, and they asked for seconds. I was ecstatic! One of them asked me what it was. At that time I didn't have a name for my creation yet. I simply looked at the empty pitcher in my hands: what had been in it was green and it looked like smoothie. So I simply said, "A green smoothie."

The message about green smoothies spread amazingly fast. I was blending nonstop, now adding other greens and apples. By the end of that day, many more people from our office complex popped in to try a green smoothie, and even our FedEx courier enjoyed it.

I continued to blend, and I started buying greens and fruit by the case. I didn't mind spending extra money and treating my friends to green smoothies, because I enjoyed hearing their overwhelmingly positive feedback. The buzz about the "green smoothie" was quickly spreading in our town and beyond.

Consuming greens in the form of green smoothies was so easy and took so little time that I naturally continued experimenting with blended greens and fruits day after day. After several weeks, I observed more improvements in my family's health. I myself felt more energized than ever before. My taste buds started to change. My occasional cravings for heavy foods, such as nuts or crackers, totally disappeared. Instead, my body was so starved for greens that for several weeks I lived almost entirely on green smoothies. Everyone in my family felt healthier, lighter, and happier.

I must admit here that the idea of blended greens was not new to me.

Ten years prior to that, in 1994, my family was studying at the Creative Health Institute in Michigan, where we learned about the extraordinary healing properties of "energy soup," blended sprouts, avocado, and apple. This soup was invented by Dr. Ann Wigmore, the pioneer of the living-foods lifestyle in the twentieth century. Although we were told countless times how exceptionally beneficial energy soup was, most of the guests at the institute were not able to eat more than a couple of spoonfuls of it, because it simply wasn't palatable.

At the same time, I was very impressed with the testimonials I heard from people who consumed it regularly, about how greatly the energy soup improved their health. When I returned home, I desperately experimented with energy soup, trying to improve the taste because I wanted my family to benefit from it. My final attempt to perfect energy soup ended one day when I heard Valya yelling to Sergei in the backyard, "Run, Sergei! Mom is making that green mush again!"

Despite all the evidence of the healing powers of energy soup, I found that, unfortunately, even some people who desperately needed and wanted it could not make themselves consume it regularly. I was amazed that ten years after being introduced to energy soup, when I had completely forgotten all about it, I suddenly came back to the very same idea of blended greens from an entirely new direction.

2 The Phenomenal Abundance of Nutrition in Greens

The most powerful . . . foods on the planet are the ones that are highest in chlorophyll. —DR. MARK SIRCUS

The majority of people living in the world today are not aware that by excluding greens from their diet they are putting themselves at risk of developing many serious health problems including diabetes, osteoporosis, depression, heart disease, obesity, and even cancer. At the very least, people who don't consume greens are destined to develop deficiencies in vitamin K and lutein simply because greens are the almost exclusive source of these two vital nutrients. A lack of vitamin K often leads to osteoporosis, anticoagulation, an increased risk of hemorrhages, nosebleeds, bleeding gums, and many other conditions. The health problems associated with lutein deficiency are cardiac disorders and poor vision. For example, have you noticed how many people in general and even little children are wearing glasses these days? When I went to school in the 1960s, we had only one girl wearing glasses in my class of thirty-five. My grandfather and my great-grandmother didn't need glasses at all and both lived to be over ninety. I believe this massive increase in poor vision is connected to a lack of greens in our diets as well as a high consumption of processed foods.

Besides lutein and vitamin K, there are many more nutrients that theoretically could be found in other foods, but in reality are readily obtained in needed amounts only from fresh greens. Greens are a rich source of important minerals such as iron, calcium, and potassium as well as many vitamins, including folate, which is abundant in greens. Greens also provide a variety of phytonutrients, or plant compounds, that protect our cells from damage, among many other effects. Dark leafy greens even contain omega-3 essential fatty acids. Calorie for calorie, dark green leafy vegetables offer the most concentrated source of nutrition of any food—most notably magnesium, the king of minerals, because it serves literally hundreds of functions in the body.

Take a look at these two molecules:

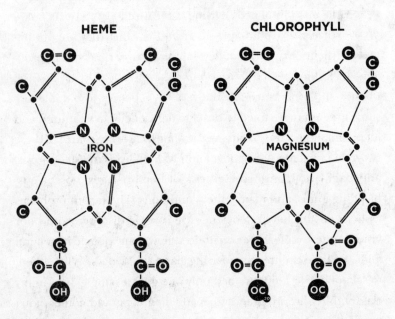

CHEMICAL FORMULAS BY KATYA KOROBKINA

The molecule on the left is a chemical representation of heme, the oxygen-carrying portion of hemoglobin, an important part of human blood. The molecule on the right is chlorophyll. As you may notice, these two molecules are almost identical in structure; the main difference is that heme contains iron in the middle, while the chlorophyll contains magnesium. I find this resemblance to be a wonderful sign of the vital importance of chlorophyll for our blood as well as for the entire body, because chlorophyll is, in essence, concentrated sunlight, a miraculous substance. And chlorophyll does indeed perform wonders of healing in a human body.

The healing powers of chlorophyll can largely be ascribed to magnesium, because the molecule of chlorophyll contains magnesium in the very center. Since people stopped consuming green vegetables on a regular basis during the Industrial Revolution, many of us have developed a serious magnesium deficiency. According to the United States Department of Agriculture (USDA), 80 percent of Americans are chronically deficient in magnesium, and magnesium deficiency is a major contributor to our epidemic of chronic and degenerative diseases, including heart disease, osteoporosis, diabetes, depression, and various autoimmune disorders.

> *Miracles in medicine would be achieved if people's*
> *magnesium deficiency was addressed instead of ignored.*
> —DR. MARK SIRCUS

Taking care of this deficiency may help with horrible "incurable" conditions that cause millions of people to suffer. Dr. Dennis Goodman, a renowned cardiologist, claims: "First and foremost, without the proper levels of magnesium in the body, we are subject to heart attacks—the number one killer of Americans."[1]

Taking magnesium can save literally hundreds of thousands

of lives yearly from a sudden, unexpected death caused by loss of heart function. It is the largest cause of natural death in the United States, causing about 325,000 adult deaths each year.[2] Like a breath of fresh air, a big burst of hope comes from the *American Journal of Clinical Nutrition:* "Researchers analyzed data from more than 88,000 women. Over the 26-year follow-up period, women whose magnesium intake was among the highest 25 percent of the subjects had a 34 percent lower adjusted risk of sudden cardiac death."[3] Dr. Liana Del Gobbo, of the Harvard School of Public Health, published a study showing magnesium can cut overall heart risk (including heart attack and stroke) by up to 22 percent.[4]

Including greens and green smoothies into daily meal plans can save millions of diabetics from suffering. Two new studies concluded that "magnesium-rich foods . . . can significantly lower the risk of developing type 2 diabetes, even in obese people."[5] Nearly 2 million Americans are currently living without an arm, leg, or foot.[6] Most losses of limbs occur as a result of type 2 diabetes, but the National Diabetic Association states: "Diabetes prevention is proven, possible, and powerful."[7]

I was not surprised. I know dozens of people who were able to reverse their symptoms by drinking green smoothies every day, even though they contain fruit. Fortunately, the same words— "prevention," "proven," "possible," and "powerful"—can also be said about most other serious conditions. Here are some other diseases and symptoms associated with magnesium deficiency:

Fibromyalgia
Cardiac arrhythmia
Osteoporosis
Arthritis
Diabetes

Back pain

Chronic fatigue syndrome

Stress and depression

Insomnia

Headaches and migraines

Ischemic heart disease (angina)

Hangover and alcoholism

Muscle cramps and spasms

Constipation

Hypertension

Asthma

Kidney stones and gall bladder stones

Dental caries

Painful menstruation and premenstrual syndrome

Processes accelerating aging (calcification)

Restless legs syndrome

Eye twitching

Sighing

Hiccups

Every organ in the body—especially the heart, muscles, and kidneys—needs magnesium. This valuable nutrient also contributes to the makeup of teeth and bones. Magnesium activates enzymes, contributes to energy production, and helps regulate calcium levels as well as copper, zinc, potassium, vitamin D, and other important nutrients in the body.

Consuming more greens is a great way to get your magnesium. Here are the greens that have the highest magnesium content:

- Swiss chard (340 g contains 275 mg magnesium)[8]
- Spinach (340 g contains 269 mg magnesium)[9]
- Stinging nettles (340 g contains 194 mg magnesium)[10]

Organically grown and wild green leafy vegetables are particularly good sources of magnesium, because conventional fields are commonly deficient in this mineral. Ocean water is the richest source of magnesium. According to scientific research, "until around 2.5 billion years ago our planet was almost completely covered by water . . . with land making up only 2 to 3 per cent of its surface."[11] That's where most magnesium came from. With the development of agriculture, the magnesium content of our soils started to drop, and today most of the farmlands are low in magnesium. The only exception are the soils in the wilderness, because nobody cuts the grass or rakes leaves in the forests and meadows. So, the magnesium from the green parts of the plants gets reabsorbed by the land every fall. For the best healing results, I recommend that you learn to add wild edibles to your green smoothies. You will notice many wild edible plant names among the ingredients in our recipes. Most of them are not sold in stores or even at farmers' markets, but each of them can easily be found in your local parks, forests, and even in your own backyard. Please be safe and first learn which wild plants are edible, and how they look before consuming them. My son Sergei has published a book, *Wild Edibles*, which contains photos and descriptions of all common edible weeds.

Just because you can explain it doesn't mean it's not still a miracle.
—TERRY PRATCHETT

Fruits are not high in magnesium, but there is a small amount in raspberries, strawberries, cantaloupe, plums, and peaches. You may add them to your green smoothies for even higher magnesium blends.

Until recently we believed that we needed to eat bananas for potassium, carrots for vitamin A, and oranges for vitamin C. Now

I invite you to look at the following facts and see for yourself how nourishing greens really are.[12] They compete and often win in nutrition over other foods. In data that comes from a most reliable source—the USDA—compare the vitamin A, potassium, and vitamin C in various 100 gram servings of food:

Vitamin A
Carrots 13,790 IU
Kale 15,376 IU

Potassium
Bananas 358 mg
Beet greens 762 mg

Vitamin C
Orange juice 50 mg
Spinach 28 mg

Of course, I don't mean that you should abandon carrots and bananas; they are healthy too, but greens are simply the winners.

I chose these examples to demonstrate the nutritional superiority of greens. Most front-line nutritionists agree that leafy greens are our most important food. Unfortunately, many people (and even some doctors) are not aware that by excluding greens from their diet, they might suffer from deficiencies, because greens are the best—and in some cases the *exclusive*—source of vital nutrients. Here is a list of nutrients that can be found almost exclusively in greens:

Vitamin K   **Folate**
Lutein   **Antioxidants**
Zeaxanthin

Let's take a closer look at each one of them.

Vitamin K

Vitamin K can be found almost exclusively in green leafy vegetables. All leafy greens have an abundance of this important, overlooked vitamin. A vitamin K deficiency has been linked to the following disorders: skin cancer; liver cancer; heavy menstrual bleeding, nosebleeds, and hemorrhaging; easy bruising; osteoporosis; hematomas; birth defects, including shortened fingers, cupped ears, flat nasal bridges, underdevelopment of the nose, mouth, and mid-face; mental retardation; and neural-tube defects.

Vitamin K2

The majority of people are not aware of the health benefits of vitamin K2, because it was discovered only within the last decade. However, we all want to have good teeth and strong bones, and vitamin K2 is critical for maintaining healthy teeth and bones.[13] A study recently published by the European Prospective Investigation into Cancer and Nutrition (EPIC) has revealed that an increased intake of vitamin K2 may reduce the risk of prostate cancer by 35 percent.[14] Besides helping to form strong teeth and bones and preventing cancer, vitamin K2 protects against heart disease, helps maintain healthy skin, promotes brain function, and supports growth and development.

Although there is almost no vitamin K2 in greens or fruit, research in Canada demonstrated that the consumption of vitamin K positively influenced the formation of vitamin K2 by human intestinal bacteria.[15] In other words, it is possible that the regular consumption of green leafy vegetables may encourage the intestinal flora in the body to produce even more vitamin K2.

Lutein and Zeaxanthin

Lutein and closely related zeaxanthin play a major role in eye health. Simply put, we need lutein to see well. Lutein is concentrated at levels up to a thousand times higher in the retina than in the rest of the body. It is also concentrated in brain tissue in both young children and adults.

Age-related macular degeneration (AMD) affects more than 1.75 million individuals in the United States. Macular degeneration is the leading cause of irreversible blindness among adults. American ophthalmological researchers conducted a study involving almost a thousand people and concluded: Those in the highest quintile of carotenoid intake had a 43 percent lower risk for AMD compared with those in the lowest quintile. Among the specific carotenoids, lutein and zeaxanthin, which are primarily obtained from dark green, leafy vegetables, were most strongly associated with a reduced risk for age-related macular degeneration.[16]

Adults are not the only ones whose vision suffers from the lutein deficiency. Researchers at the University of Georgia have discovered that lutein deficiency may lead to poor visual performance in healthy young people, especially those exposed to glaring light conditions. After supplementing the diets of a group of young people with lutein and zeaxanthin each day for six months, all participants demonstrated improved visual performance.[17]

Because the human body cannot synthesize lutein, we need to get lutein from food. The average American consumes 0.8–1.0 milligram daily.[18] No recommended daily amount has been set for lutein or zeaxanthin. However, the American Optometric Association recommends 10 milligrams a day of lutein and 2 milligrams a day of zeaxanthin.

Here is a list of some foods with lutein plus zeaxanthin (milligrams per 100 gram serving):

Kale 39.6	Corn 0.9
Spinach 15.7	Egg 0.4
Dandelion greens 13.6	Nectarines 0.1
Turnip greens 11.9	Papaya 0.08
Collard greens 10.8	Cauliflower 0.03
Zucchini squash 2.1	Apples 0.03
Broccoli 1.4	

As you can see, dark leafy greens are our *only* realistic source of lutein. Its content in other foods is so minute that in order to consume enough lutein, you would have to eat 42 eggs or 73 pounds of apples in one day.

Folate

Humans cannot synthesize folate; therefore, folate has to be supplied through the diet to meet daily requirements. It is important to understand that there is a big difference between folate and folic acid. Folate is a general term for a group of water-soluble B vitamins, also known as B9. Folic acid refers to the oxidized synthetic compound used in dietary supplements and food fortification.

If you look for sources of folate online, you may discover a wide variety of foods, such as breads and pastas, listed as good sources of folic acid. Remember the difference pointed out above—these foods are merely fortified with synthetic folic acid. Regular consumption of them can lead to excessive intake of folic acid. There is scientific evidence that accumulation of large amounts of this artificial compound could have negative effects on health, such as rash, diarrhea, dizziness, fatigue, and gas.[19]

Although folate deficiency is a prevalent phenomenon world-wide, we do not need synthetic folic acid supplements to meet our daily folate requirements. Folate is abundant in all green vegetables. You can easily get your daily recommendation of 500–600 mcg. of folate by adding a quart of green smoothie to your everyday menu.

Essential for numerous bodily functions, folate:

- aids the complete development of red blood cells;
- reduces blood levels of homocysteine, a toxic by-product of amino-acid metabolism that may promote atherosclerosis and osteoporosis;
- supports cell production, especially in the skin;
- helps prevent osteoporosis-related bone fractures;
- is necessary for fertility in both men and women;
- helps prevent dementias, including Alzheimer's disease;
- supports nervous-system function;
- helps prevent neural-tube defects in newborns (so women of childbearing age must be sure to have an adequate intake prior to and during pregnancy).

Antioxidants

Antioxidants are chemicals that interact with and neutralize free radicals, thus preventing them from causing cell damage. Antioxidants are also known as "free-radical scavengers." Because of their high content of antioxidants, green leafy vegetables are one of the best cancer-preventing foods.

Today's cancer statistics are very depressing. In 2013, almost 1,600 Americans died from cancer each day. Cancer remains the second most common cause of death in the United States, accounting for nearly one out of every four deaths.[20] However, despite these sad numbers, there is a real change happening already. According to the American Institute for Cancer Research, carotenoids in dark green leafy vegetables may protect against:

- Cancers of the mouth, pharynx, and larynx
- Certain types of breast cancer
- Skin cancer
- Lung cancer
- Stomach cancer
- Pancreatic cancer
- Colorectal cancer[21]

Similar conclusions come from Asian scientists: Varieties of greens from the brassica family are sources of important antioxidants and anti-inflammatories related to the prevention of chronic diseases associated with oxidative stress, such as in cancer and coronary artery disease.[22]

These and many other scientific research studies make complete sense. If greens are the most nutritious food on our planet, then it is logical that we need to continue to eat greens on a daily basis, as we have done throughout our history. Living a long and healthy life is everyone's birthright, and greens are definitely the most efficient way to accomplish this.

My son Stephan, who had his tonsils removed many years ago, now drinks green smoothies daily and enjoys good health. Several times a week he rides fifty miles on his bicycle. Stephan has just celebrated his fortieth birthday. My quest for natural health started almost forty years ago. Sadly, more than 530,000 children under fifteen have their tonsils removed surgically every year just in the United States.[23]

I strongly believe that the easiest and most effective way to prevent one's health problems starts with the daily consumption of freshly blended green smoothies.

Similarly, fruits and other vegetables contain a number of essential vitamins, nutrients, and minerals. When mixed in with greens, they help pack smoothies with a delicious and nutritious punch. Just take a look at the eye-popping nutrients found in your favorite greens, fruits, and vegetables.

Nutrient Content of Greens, Fruits, and Vegetables

VITAMINS	FOUND IN	FUNCTIONS
A	All greens, most vegetables (with the highest content in sweet potatoes, carrots, and squash), and most fruits, especially mangos, apricots, peaches, papayas, cantaloupe, and oranges.	Essential for the growth and development of cells; keeps skin healthy; supports the immune and reproduction systems; vital for vision.
C	All greens, all fruits (with the highest content in guavas, oranges, and kiwis), and all vegetables, especially bell peppers and broccoli.	As an antioxidant, fights off free radicals in the body; wards off inflammation, infections, and viruses; helps form collagen, the main structural protein in connective tissue; essential for healthy bones, teeth, gums, and blood vessels; helps the body absorb iron; accelerates the healing process; improves cognitive function; strengthens the immune system; protects against heart attacks and strokes, which leads to better vascular health and increases longevity; is important in preventing Alzheimer's disease, autoimmune problems, and atherosclerosis.

VITAMINS	FOUND IN	FUNCTIONS
E (alpha-tocopherol)	Greens, sprouts, kiwis, mangos, apricots, tomatoes, avocados, bell peppers, asparagus, pumpkin, parsnips, and broccoli.	As a powerful antioxidant, protects cell membranes against damage caused by free radicals; prevents the oxidation of LDL cholesterol, which keeps the free radicals clear of the body's blood vessels; essential for maintenance of skeletal, cardiac, and smooth muscle; assists in the formation of red blood cells; and positively influences immune health.
K	Greens and green vegetables.	Maintains adequate blood clotting and protects against osteoporosis, arterial calcification, cardiovascular disease, varicose veins, prostate cancer, lung cancer, liver cancer, leukemia, and a number of brain health problems, including dementia.
B1 (thiamine)	Dark greens such as kale and lettuces, tomatoes, green peas, squash, asparagus, cucumbers, pineapples, oranges, cantaloupe, watermelon, grapefruits, and many other fruits and vegetables.	Helps convert food into energy needed for healthy skin, hair, nerves, muscles, and brain.
B2 (riboflavin)	Watercress, beet greens, sweet potato leaves, spinach, other greens, avocados, bell peppers, passion fruit, durians, tamarinds, longans, cherimoya, and plums.	Helps convert food into energy; needed for healthy skin, hair, blood, nails, eyes, lips, mouth, and tongue; fights fatigue; protects against cancer. (Chronic alcoholics and pregnant women are susceptible to a deficiency of this vitamin.)
B3 (niacin)	Cilantro, borage, parsley, spinach, tomatoes, bell peppers, tomatillos, asparagus, and okra.	Helps convert food into energy; essential for the digestive and nervous systems, blood-cell protection, and brain function.

VITAMINS	FOUND IN	FUNCTIONS
B5 (pantothenic acid)	Endive, watercress, cilantro, arugula, turnip greens, cucumbers, broccoli, celery, pumpkin, radishes, bell peppers, avocados, grapefruit, water-melon, blackberries, cranberries, and raspberries.	Helps convert food into energy; aids in the production of many important compounds such as fatty acids, cholesterol, neurotransmitters, steroid hormones, and hemoglobin.
B6 (pyridoxine)	Spinach, turnip greens, kale, bell peppers, green peas, yams, broccoli, asparagus, avoca-dos, bananas, pineapples, straw-berries, figs, and watermelon.	Aids in lowering levels of homocysteine and may reduce the risk of heart disease; helps convert tryptophan to niacin and serotonin, a neurotransmit-ter that plays key roles in sleep, appetite, and mood; helps red blood cells influence cognitive abilities and the function of the immune system.
B7 (biotin)	Swiss chard, romaine lettuce, bananas, avocados, onions, cucumbers, cauliflower, black-berries, blueberries, and strawberries.	Essential for metabolism; processes every type of food ingested, including carbohydrates, protein, and fat; helps convert food into energy and synthe-size glucose; necessary for cell growth; helps strengthen hair and nails.
B9 (folate)	Spinach, turnip greens, parsley, mustard greens, lettuces, collards, all other greens, beets, okra, parsnips, green peas, cauli-flower, bell peppers, avocados, oranges, papaya, strawber-ries, and raspber-ries.	Vital for new cell creation; helps prevent brain and spine birth defects when consumed early in pregnancy; essential for women of child-bearing age; can lower levels of homocysteine; may reduce heart disease risk.

VITAMINS	FOUND IN	FUNCTIONS
Choline	Celery, parsley, cilantro, spinach, mustard greens, herbs, beets, asparagus, avocados, blackberries, dates, peaches, and pears.	Helps make and release acetylcholine, a neurotransmitter that aids in many nerve and brain activities; plays a role in metabolizing and transporting fats.
Betaine	Spinach and beets.	Helps the liver process fats; plays a role in reducing blood levels of homocysteine; boosts muscle protein synthesis.

MINERALS	FOUND IN	GOOD FOR
Calcium	Stinging nettles, spinach, kale, turnips, collards and other greens, garlic, okra, dates, blackberries, oranges, kumquats, prickly pears, mulberries, apricots, figs, and kiwis.	Builds and protects bones and teeth; slows down the loss of bone density during aging; helps with muscle contraction; plays a role in hormone secretion and enzyme activation.
Chromium	Spinach, lettuces, basil, other greens, broccoli, beets, tomatoes, apples, and bananas.	Enhances the activity of insulin; helps maintain normal blood glucose levels; needed to free energy from glucose.
Copper	Kale, turnip greens, chard, spinach, cilantro, other greens, avocados, asparagus, radicchio, radishes, squash, okra, blackberries, guavas, and dates.	Copper is involved in the formation of red blood cells, the absorption and utilization of iron, the metabolism of cholesterol and glucose, and the synthesis and release of life-sustaining proteins and enzymes. These enzymes in turn produce cellular energy and regulate nerve transmission, blood clotting, and oxygen transport. Copper stimulates the immune system to fight infections, to repair injured tissues, and to promote healing. Copper also helps to neutralize free radicals, which can cause severe damage to cells.

MINERALS	FOUND IN	GOOD FOR
Fluoride	Lettuce, celery, cucumbers, carrots, cabbage, onions, radishes, strawberries, peaches, bananas, plums, and watermelon.	Encourages strong bone formation.
Iron	Spinach, collards, parsley, purslane, all greens, pumpkin, red cabbage, okra, carrots, mulberries, pomegranates, currants, persimmons, and watermelon.	Makes up part of hemoglobin molecule found in red blood cells; needed for chemical reactions in the body and for making amino acids, collagen, neurotransmitters, and hormones.
Magnesium	Chard, dock, beet greens, spinach, all greens, avocados, artichokes, beets, raspberries, bananas, figs, strawberries, plums, and apples.	Required for many chemical reactions in the body; works with calcium in muscle contraction and relaxation process, blood clotting, and regulation of blood pressure; keeps nerves and muscles strong; helps build bones and teeth.
Manganese	Lettuce, spinach, endive, arugula, broccoli, kale, collard greens, dandelion greens, mustard greens, all greens, blueberries, pineapples, blackberries, strawberries, and raspberries.	Aids bone formation; helps metabolize amino acids, cholesterol, and carbohydrates.
Phosphorus	Watercress, parsley, leeks, garlic, celery, tomatoes, durians.	Essential to DNA and RNA; helps build and protect bones and teeth; aids in converting food into energy; component of phospholipids, which carry lipids in the blood and help shuttle nutrients into and out of cells; helps maintain acid-base balance.

MINERALS	FOUND IN	GOOD FOR
Potassium	Beet greens, purslane, watercress, spinach, all greens, radishes, tomatoes, avocados, papayas, melons, guavas, peaches, apricots, dates, raisins, figs, coconut, bananas, nectarines, and other fruits.	Keeps fluids balanced in blood and tissue; helps maintain a steady heartbeat and send nerve impulses, which are needed for muscle contractions; aids in lowering blood pressure.
Selenium	Spinach, amaranth leaves, other greens, asparagus, chia seeds, bananas, mangos, grapefruit, lemons, and cantaloupe.	As an antioxidant, neutralizes unstable molecules that can damage cells; helps regulate thyroid hormone activity.
Sodium	Swiss chard, beet greens, celery, watercress, other greens, turnips, carrots, beets, bell peppers, guavas, passion fruit, honeydew, and pineapples.	Sends nerve impulses required to contract the body's muscles; attracts and holds water to help maintain the liquid portion of the blood.
Zinc	Swiss chard, asparagus, pumpkin, avocados, apricots, peaches, pomegranates, plums, bananas, figs, blackberries, raspberries, and dates.	Helps form about 100 enzymes in the body; supports healthy immune system; is necessary to synthesize DNA; is essential for wound healing; supports the healthy growth and development of the body during adolescence, childhood, and pregnancy; frees vitamin A from storage in the liver; important in influencing taste, smell, and wound healing; may delay the progression of age-related macular degeneration when taken with certain antioxidants.

OTHER NUTRIENTS	FOUND IN	GOOD FOR
Fiber	All greens, artichokes, peas, broccoli, avocados, raspberries, blackberries, pears, and all fruits.	Optimizes the function of the friendly bacteria in the intestine; reduces constipation; reduces spikes in blood sugar after a high-carb meal; can reduce blood cholesterol levels; can help people lose weight.
Flavonoids	Spinach, chard, other greens, colored bell peppers, tomatoes, okra, garlic, strawberries, blueberries, blackberries, oranges, lemons, peaches, nectarines, mangos, papayas, other colorful berries and fruits, dill, turmeric, thyme, and most other spices.	As superantioxidants, increase bodily health in many ways; promote the formation of strong cells and the suppression of poor cellular growth, delivering an anticarcinogenic effect; contribute to good heart health; combat atherosclerosis as well as conditions like Alzheimer's disease; help hemoglobin in red blood cells and myoglobin in muscle cells ferry oxygen throughout the body; needed for making amino acids, collagen, neurotransmitters, and hormones.

3 Your A–Z Nutrient Prescription

The food you eat can be either the safest and most powerful form of medicine or the slowest form of poison. —ANN WIGMORE

In my experience, people often face a dilemma when they first join the green-smoothie revolution. Which greens, fruits, and vegetables should I throw into the blender to get the right nutrients for me? As the chart in the previous chapter demonstrates, different foods contain different vitamins and minerals. Consider this A–Z Nutrient Prescription, then, your handy go-to reference guide for choosing the best ingredients with the most effective nutrients for battling everything from minor colds and aches and pains to chronic conditions and debilitating diseases.

Aloe Vera

Aloe vera is a medicinal plant full of nutritional benefits. I love to add a one-inch piece of aloe vera leaf to my smoothies, but only a couple times a month, because it is a strong medicinal plant and consuming it too much and too often may produce diarrhea.

At the same time, aloe vera contains over two hundred active components, including vitamins, minerals, amino acids, enzymes, polysaccharide, and fatty acids.

Aloe vera contains vitamins A, C, and E plus the minerals zinc and selenium. Antioxidants present in aloe vera help combat free radicals in the body. It also contains vitamins B1, B2, B3, B5, and B6, along with choline, calcium, magnesium, zinc, manganese, chromium, and selenium.

In the sap of the leaves, phenolic compounds called anthraquinones are located; they have stimulating effects on the bowels and antibiotic properties. They also help with absorption from the gastrointestinal tract and have antimicrobial and painkilling effects.

Amaranth Greens

Amaranth leaves come from a bushy perennial wild edible. Amaranth greens are packed with carbohydrates, proteins, vitamins K, A, C, B2, B6, and folate, all of which boost energy in the body. High dietary fiber content (three times that of wheat) in the greens aids digestive health and reduces constipation.

Amaranth leaves are an excellent source of manganese, iron, copper, calcium, magnesium, potassium, and phosphorus, necessary for maintaining proper mineral balance in the body.

Amaranth greens and grains have been noted for reducing the risk of Alzheimer's disease and dementia.

Apples

Apples are a great source of soluble and insoluble fiber. Soluble fiber, such as pectin, helps prevent cholesterol buildup in the lining of blood-vessel walls, which in turn reduces risk for heart disease and atherosclerosis. Phytonutrients in apples can help regulate blood sugar. Apples also contain iron, potassium, folate, calcium, phosphorus, and vitamins A and C. It is a good idea to eat apples with the skin on, as most of the vitamin C content is located under the skin.

Apricots

Apricots contain high levels of vitamin A, which benefits the eyes, skin, hair, and various glands. Vitamin A also helps fight off infections by keeping the immune system strong. Just one fresh or dried apricot provides the daily recommended allowance of vitamin A. In addition, apricots also contain vitamins C, E, K, B6, and B17, which are believed to have cancer-fighting properties.

Arugula

Arugula (a cruciferous vegetable, i.e., in the same plant family as cauliflower, cabbage, and broccoli) is a good source of calcium, iron, manganese, copper, potassium, folate, and vitamins A, C, and K. The primary benefits of arugula leaves come from their phytochemical content. Regular consumption of arugula helps to prevent most types of cancer. Some of the phytochemicals, such as glucosinolates and sulforaphanes, are responsible for stimulating enzymes that help the body cleanse itself of toxins and potential carcinogens. Vitamin A contains powerful antioxidants. Carotenes, for example, can protect against sun damage, heart disease, and cancer. Antioxidants in arugula support the well-being of cellular function. Arugula is a rich source of chlorophyll, which cleanses and energizes the blood. It helps bring large amounts of oxygen to all parts of the body and suppresses viruses and harmful bacteria. Chlorophyll also supports healthy skin and helps limit the effect of potential carcinogens.

Avocados

Avocados contain oleic acid, a monounsaturated fat that may help to lower cholesterol. Avocados are a good source of potassium, a mineral that helps regulate blood pressure. Avocados are rich in other essential nutrients, including fiber, B vitamins, vitamins E, C, and K, folate, and magnesium. Avocado pits are also rich in soluble fiber, which can help to control cholesterol.

Bananas

Bananas are one of our best sources of potassium, an essential mineral for maintaining normal blood pressure and heart function. A banana a day may help to protect against atherosclerosis and promote bone health. Potassium, one of the most important electrolytes, which helps regulate heart function as well as fluid balance, may counteract the increased urinary calcium loss caused by the high-salt diets, thus helping to prevent bones from thinning out at a fast rate. Bananas also contain vitamins A, K, C, and E, folate, choline, calcium, magnesium, phosphorus, sodium, selenium, fluoride, and iron.

Bananas have long been recognized for their antacid effects, which protect against stomach ulcers and ulcer damage. In addition, bananas contain pectin, a soluble fiber that can help normalize movement through the digestive tract and ease constipation.

Basil

Basil is a good source of vitamin A, which helps to prevent damage to the cells by free radicals. Also present in basil, magnesium helps the heart and blood vessels to relax, improving blood flow. Other nutrients found in basil include iron, calcium, potassium, and vitamin C. An array of flavonoids exist in basil, which help to protect cells and chromosomes from damage. One of the primary medicinal uses of basil comes from (E)-BCP, or (E)-beta-caryophyllene, a natural anti-inflammatory compound. (E)-BCP found in basil may offer an alternative to medical marijuana, because it has the same anti-inflammatory effects without the mental and neurological side effects. (E)-BCP in basil is believed to combat bowel inflammation and rheumatoid arthritis.

Antioxidants in basil make it a healthy booster for the immune system. Fresh basil leaves have antibacterial properties and can actually be used to clean surfaces of infectious disease. Basil leaves applied topically to wounds may also eliminate bacterial infections. Ingesting basil as a culinary herb or supplement can also give the body an ability to combat viral infections, including colds, flu, and herpes-family viruses.

Bee Pollen

Bee pollen contains twenty-two amino acids; it is approximately 40 percent protein.

It is amazingly rich in many vitamins: A (carotene), B1, B2, B3, B5, B6, B12, C, D, E, F, H, K, PP, folate, choline, inositol, and rutin.

Bee pollen also is rich in minerals: calcium, phosphorus, potassium, iron, copper, iodine, zinc, sulfur, sodium, chlorine, magnesium, manganese, molybdenum, selenium, boron, silica, and titanium.

Bee pollen has an ability to strengthen immunity, counteract the effects of radiation and chemical toxins (which are the two most severe stressors to your immune system), and generate optimal health and vitality.

However, bee pollen is the food of young bees, and as such strict vegans exclude it from their diet; for this reason in our recipes we say "optional" in parentheses. Bee pollen is available at many health food stores.

Beet Greens

Beet greens contain very large amounts of vitamin K, an important element that aids in blood clotting and plays a role in fighting diseases that afflict the elderly, such as Alzheimer's disease and osteoporosis. Vitamin K works alongside calcium to boost the strength of bones. Vitamin K is also known to provide relief from pregnancy symptoms like morning sickness and menstrual conditions like excessive bleeding.

Vitamin A is found in large amounts in beet greens. Vitamin A brings a wide range of health benefits to the body, such as the maintenance of good vision. Vitamin A strengthens the immune system. This vitamin stimulates antibodies and white blood cells, which protect against infections. Studies have shown that vitamin A can play a role in cancer prevention. If you regularly consume vitamin A–rich plants like beet greens, you have a lower risk of developing cancer than if you get your vitamin A from animal products. For pregnant women, vitamin A helps in embryonic development. A vitamin-A compound, beta-carotene, is an antioxidant that can fight the aging process and other effects of free radicals in the body.

Birch Tree Leaves

Birch leaves are rich in vitamins C, E, PP, and carotene. Birch leaves are very rich in flavonoids, which can destroy free radicals.

Tannins that are abundant in birch leaves have antibacterial and anti-inflammatory properties. Juice of young birch leaves has been used for treating inflammations and infections of the urinary tract, edema, and kidney stones.

Blackberries

Blackberries are rich in antioxidant vitamins A and C. Possibly the most promising benefit from consuming blackberries is the substantial quantity of phenolic acids, which are antioxidant compounds known as potent anticarcinogenic agents. Medical research shows the regular consumption of blackberries may benefit those with pleurisy, lung inflammation, thrombosis, cancer, endotoxin shock, cardiovascular disease, diabetes, and age-related cognitive decline.

Blueberries

According to the USDA Human Nutritional Center, blueberries rank number one in antioxidant benefits compared to forty other fruits and vegetables. Antioxidants help neutralize harmful free radicals that can lead to cancer and age-related diseases. The total antioxidant capacity of blueberries is twice as much as spinach and three times as much as oranges. This extraordinary fruit is also rich in pectin, a soluble fiber that has been shown to be effective in lowering cholesterol. In addition, blueberries have also been shown to be beneficial for diabetics, as they are a low-glycemic food that helps slow down the absorption of sugars in the bloodstream.

Bok Choy

Bok choy is known to aid in healthy digestion. It is an excellent source of folate and high in vitamin A, vitamin C, vitamin B6, beta-carotene, calcium, potassium, and dietary fiber. Bok choy contains some powerful antioxidants. The beta-carotene in bok choy can help to reduce the risk of cataracts and certain cancers.

Borage

Fresh borage has high levels of vitamin C, a powerful natural antioxidant that helps to remove harmful free radicals from the body. Vitamin C is known to boost the immune system and heal wounds, and it has antiviral effects. Borage contains very high levels of vitamin A and carotenes, which are powerful flavonoid antioxidants. Together, they protect against free radicals. Vitamin A is essential for vision and is also required for maintaining healthy mucus membranes and skin. Consumption of natural foods rich in vitamin A and carotenes is known to protect from lung and oral-cavity cancers.

Borage has a good amount of minerals like iron, calcium, potassium, manganese, copper, zinc, and magnesium. Potassium is an important component of cell and body fluids and helps control heart rate and blood pressure. Iron is an important component of hemoglobin inside the red blood cells; it determines the oxygen-carrying capacity of the blood. Borage is a good source of B-complex vitamins and is particularly rich in vitamin B3 (niacin). Niacin helps lower LDL cholesterol levels in the body. In addition, it has vitamins B1, B2, B6, and folate in adequate amounts. These vitamins function as cofactors in the enzymatic metabolism inside the body. Naturopathic doctors often use borage for regulating metabolism and the hormonal system and for treating PMS symptoms, menopause symptoms, hot flashes, colds, bronchitis, respiratory infections, and inflammation.

Cantaloupe

Cantaloupe is extremely high in vitamins A and C. A cup of cantaloupe, for instance, provides 103 percent of the recommended daily amount of vitamin A and 112 percent of the recommended daily amount of vitamin C. Vitamin A is known to reduce the risk of developing cataracts. Vitamin C is critical for good immune function. It also stimulates white cells to fight infection by directly killing many bacteria and viruses. In addition, cantaloupe contains good levels of B vitamins as well as folate and potassium.

Carrot-Top Greens

Carrot tops are rich in protein, vitamins, and minerals. They contain up to six times more vitamin C than carrot roots, and several times more than lemons. They are an excellent source of calcium and chlorophyll, which is credited with therapeutic properties to clean up the blood, lymph nodes, and adrenal glands from poisons and to strengthen bones and muscles.

Carrot tops are rich in potassium and vitamin K, which lowers blood pressure, maintains normal metabolism, and prevents osteoporosis and heart disease. The Greek physician Pedanius Dioscorides included carrot tops in the list of six hundred species of medicinal plants that are effective in the treatment of cancer.

Juice of the leaves can be used as an antiseptic mouthwash. It is enough to chew a sprig of carrot leaf to get rid of bad breath, bleeding gums, and sores. Carrot tops have strong antiseptic properties.

They can be mixed with honey to disinfect wounds.

Carrot tops contain significant amounts of porphyrins that stimulate the pituitary gland and lead to increased production of sex hormones.

If you suffer from insomnia, you can apply carrot tops to the back of your head. A poultice with carrot tops wrapped around the legs for a few hours relieves pain from varicose veins.

Carrot tops are a very good source of folate, which is very useful for the nervous system and brain. They also contain a lot of iron, magnesium, potassium, calcium, and iodine.

Cayenne Pepper

Cayenne pepper is an excellent source of vitamin A. The hotness produced by cayenne is caused by its high concentration of a substance called capsaicin. Capsaicin has been widely studied for its pain-reducing effects, its cardiovascular benefits, and its ability to help prevent ulcers. Capsaicin also effectively opens and drains congested nasal passages.

Celery

Celery contains vitamin C and several other active compounds that promote health, including coumarins, which may be useful in cancer prevention, and phthalides, which can both lower cholesterol and help relax the muscles around arteries, allowing those vessels to dilate. With more space inside the arteries, the blood can flow at a lower blood pressure. Celery ranks as a very good source of potassium and a good source of calcium and magnesium, and increased intake of these minerals has also been associated with reduced blood pressure.

Cherries

Many of the health benefits of cherries are related to the natural chemical that gives them their color, anthocyanin. Anthocyanins are used by the body to produce essential amino acids. As antioxidants, anthocyanins protect the cells of the body from the damaging, aging, and disease-producing effects of oxygen, nitrogen, and ultraviolet radiation. Anthocyanins are also natural pain relievers and anti-inflammatories. Regular cherry consumption can prevent short- and long-term damage to muscles. This makes cherries a great food for pre- and post-workout snacks.

Cherries also contain high levels of melatonin. Research has shown that people who have heart attacks demonstrate low melatonin levels. Besides being an antioxidant, melatonin helps regulate sleep and wake cycles and has also been shown to be important for the functioning of the immune system.

Chia Seeds

Chia seeds are a good source of calcium, phosphorus, manganese, and zinc and are extremely rich in omega-3 essential fatty acids and easy-to-digest protein. They have been proven to be a great power food with anti-inflammatory properties.

Chia seeds have been getting national attention from ultrarunners and endurance athletes, because they are able to absorb more than twelve times their weight in water. Their ability to hold on to water allows hydration to be prolonged. Chia seeds help to retain moisture, making the utilization of body fluids and the maintenance of electrolyte balance more efficient. Chia seeds are an effective muscle and tissue builder.

Chia seeds also have significant benefits for diabetics, because they have the ability to stabilize blood sugar and are known to help in losing extra weight.

Cilantro

Cilantro (coriander) is rich in antioxidants and dietary fiber, which help reduce LDL, or "bad cholesterol," and increase HDL, or "good cholesterol," levels. Cilantro contains many essential volatile oils. The leaves and stem tips are rich in numerous antioxidant polyphenolic flavonoids. The herb is a good source of minerals like potassium, calcium, manganese, iron, and magnesium. Potassium is an important component of cell and body fluids that helps control heart rate and blood pressure. Iron is essential for red blood cell production. Manganese is used by the body as a cofactor for the antioxidant enzyme superoxide dismutase. Cilantro is also rich in many vital vitamins, including B2, B3, folate, A, beta-carotene, and C, which are essential for optimum health. Vitamin C is a powerful natural antioxidant. Vitamin A is required for maintaining healthy mucus membranes and skin and is also essential for vision. Consuming natural foods rich in vitamin A and flavonoids (carotenes) helps protect the body from lung and oral-cavity cancers. Cilantro also provides vitamin K, which is important for bone mass building. It also has an established role in the treatment of Alzheimer's disease by limiting neuronal damage in the brain. Recent research shows cilantro's ability to bind to heavy metals and help remove them from the body.

Cinnamon

Cinnamon is said to regulate blood sugar. Cinnamon also helps lower LDL cholesterol, remedies and prevents yeast infections, has anticlotting properties, and boosts cognitive functions and memory.

Coconut

Coconut (young coconut meat and water) is an excellent source of manganese, phosphorus, and potassium. Coconut also contains protein, calcium, niacin (B3), folate, iron, magnesium, and zinc, among other essential minerals. Fresh young coconut meat is noted for being a great source for dietary fiber, which prevents constipation. Coconut also helps build muscle bulk, cure sore throats, and relieve stomach ulcers; helps diabetes by protecting against "insulin resistance;"[1] helps kidney problems; and produces healthy, radiant skin. In addition, coconut water hydrates the body by replenishing electrolytes.

Collard Greens

Packed with nutrition, collard greens are loaded with anticancer properties and are an excellent source of vitamins B6 and C, carotenes, chlorophyll, and manganese. One cup of collard greens provides more than 70 percent of the recommended daily allowance of vitamin C. Collard greens are also a very good source of fiber, minerals—iron, copper, and calcium—and vitamins B1, B2, and E.

Collard greens may have the most cholesterol-lowering ability of all the commonly eaten cruciferous vegetables. They contain phytonutrients called glucosinolates, which can help activate detoxification enzymes and regulate their activity. As an excellent source of vitamin C, beta-carotene, and manganese, and a good source of vitamin E and zinc, collard greens provide us with extensive antioxidant support, which helps lower oxidative stress in cells, a risk factor for the development of most cancer types. Collard is an excellent source of vitamin K and a very good source of omega-3 fatty acids, two top anti-inflammatory nutrients that may reverse blood-vessel damage.

Cranberries

Cranberries are very high in vitamins C, A, E, K, B6, and B5 as well as manganese. Cranberries also have extremely high levels of flavonoids and antioxidants, and antioxidants combat the oxidative stress due to free radicals in a great many diseases, including cancer, heart and vascular disease, diabetes, inflammation, and neurological disorders. Premature aging and diseases of the elderly, such as macular degeneration, are thought to result from oxidative damage to cells as well. Cranberries are also great for curing and preventing urinary-tract infections.

Cremini Mushrooms

Cremini mushrooms are small, button-shaped, rich brown mushrooms, which are in fact mini-Portabellas. Cremini mushrooms are an excellent source of selenium, which helps to fight cancer. Other minerals in cremini mushrooms are copper, potassium, phosphorus, selenium, iron, calcium, and zinc. Potassium is the mineral that brings down your blood pressure and reduces your risk of stroke. Cremini mushrooms are a good source of vitamins E, D, B1, B2, B3, and B5.

Cremini mushrooms contain tryptophan, which is an essential amino acid. Tryptophan affects the neurotransmitter serotonin.

This is the component that allows you to control your sleep patterns and mood swings.

Cremini mushrooms have a high amount of a powerful antioxidant L-ergothioneine. This ingredient is able to protect cells from mutating and from UV and radiation damage and to detox the liver, as well as improve eye health, reproductive health, and lung health.

Cremini mushrooms also contain anti-inflammatory properties that can effectively regulate inflammation in the heart, joints, organs, and tissues, making them especially good for those who suffer from arthritis, heart disease, asthma, fibromyalgia, and chronic fatigue syndrome.

Cucumbers

Cucumbers contain vitamin C and caffeic acid, both of which help soothe skin irritations and reduce swelling. Cucumbers' hard skin is rich in fiber and contains a variety of beneficial minerals, including silica, potassium, and magnesium. Cucumbers are a very good source of potassium, an important intracellular electrolyte. Potassium also helps reduce blood pressure and heart rates by countering the effects of sodium. Cucumbers contain unique antioxidants in good ratios. These compounds protect against free radicals that play a role in aging. Cucumbers have a mild diuretic property due to their high water content, which is helpful in checking weight loss and high blood pressure. Cucumbers have a relatively high amount of vitamin K, which has a potential role in the increase of bone mass. They also have an established role in treating Alzheimer's disease by limiting neuronal damage in the brain.

Dandelion Greens

Dandelion greens are beneficial in a number of ways. They help improve bone health, combat liver disorders, diabetes, acne, cancer, jaundice, and anemia. Dandelion leaves contain beta-carotene, vitamins B1, B2, B5, B6, B12, C, and E as well as minerals like iron, calcium, potassium, phosphorus, magnesium, and zinc.

Dates

Dates are high in vitamins C, B1, B2, B3, B5, and A, as well as folate, calcium, magnesium, phosphorus, potassium, and natural sugars. The sugars in dates are paired with dietary fiber, a wonderful combination that makes dates a great energy food. Dates are rich in soluble and insoluble fiber. The sugar-fiber combination ensures that your body will have clean, even-burning fuel, no matter what kind of exercise you engage in. Dates are rich in potassium and low in sodium. Research has shown that a higher intake of potassium (about 400 milligrams) can cut the risk of stroke by 40 percent. Other important minerals include copper, iron, and manganese. Dates have a dense concentration of phenol antioxidants. Another key health benefit of dates is their ability to lower undesirable LDL cholesterol.

Dill Weed

Dill is loaded with antioxidants, which kill free radicals in the body and help prevent cancer. Dill is loaded with vitamins A and C, copper, potassium, calcium, manganese, iron, and magnesium. Dill provides great relief to those suffering from diarrhea, dysentery, and menstrual disorders. In this regard it is similar to garlic in preventing bacterial overgrowth. Dill also helps in the secretion of bile and digestive juices, which further aid digestion. Dill also helps stimulate the appetite.

Dock Greens

Dock is a wild green that can be used in any recipe where we traditionally use kale, spinach, or other greens. When someone shows you this plant, you most likely will recognize it as commonly found in your backyard and in parks and gardens.

Dock is high in vitamins C and A, protein, magnesium, calcium, phosphorus, potassium, manganese, iron, and selenium. These greens contain the highest amount of magnesium that I was able to find in different greens, which makes dock valuable for diabetics, people suffering with fibromyalgia, migraines, leg cramps, and other conditions associated with magnesium deficiency.

Douglas Fir Needles

The vitamin C content in Douglas fir needles is extremely high, but exhibits seasonal variation within the range of 100–350 milligrams per 100 grams of fresh weight. Oils in Douglas fir have strong antimicrobial effects against bacteria, fungi, and worms. *Warning:* This is a medicinal plant. Use only a handful of needles at a time and only young, light-green needles. Douglas fir needles reduce or eliminate phlegm and stimulate lung health. They have been used traditionally as cold and cough remedies. Douglas fir needle extract is also used to treat infections, stimulate metabolism, and for cosmetics and skin care.

Durians

A great source of minerals and vitamins, durians are also an excellent source of many health-benefiting B-complex vitamins, including B1, B2, B3, B5, and B6. All the B vitamins are water-soluble and are excreted from the body fairly quickly. That is why these vitamins are essential and need to be replenished on a daily basis. Durians also contain a high amount of minerals like manganese, copper, iron, and magnesium. Manganese is used by the body as a cofactor for the antioxidant enzyme superoxide dismutase, and the body requires copper and iron for red blood cell formation. Also found in durians are high levels of the essential amino acid tryptophan (also known as "nature's sleeping pill"), which in the body metabolizes into serotonin and melatonin, neurochemicals that have important functions like sleep induction and, in certain cases, the treatment of epilepsy.

Endive

Endive is very low in calories (about 95 percent water and 7.5 calories per cup) and high in nutrition. It is an excellent source of vitamins A and C, fiber, calcium, chlorine, iron, phosphorus, potassium, and sulfur. Endive is beneficial for such conditions as acne, asthma, anemia, cancer, constipation, and liver and gall bladder problems.

Fennel Greens

Fennel is an excellent source of vitamin C, folate, potassium, manganese, niacin, phosphorous, calcium, magnesium, iron, copper, and dietary fiber. With only 27 calories per cup, fennel is one of the best antioxidants and anti-inflammatory foods on the planet.

The phytonutrients in fennel—rutin, quercetin, and anethole—have been found to reduce inflammation and help prevent cancer.

The volatile oils in fennel promote digestion and absorption of food by increasing the secretion of digestive enzymes in the stomach, which makes fennel a great food for acid reflux.

Figs

Fresh figs, especially black mission, are high in polyphenolic flavonoid antioxidants such as carotenes, lutein, tannins, and chlorogenic acid.

Fresh figs contain adequate levels of some of the antioxidant vitamins such as vitamin A, E, and K, which help scavenge harmful free radicals from the body and thereby protect us from cancers, diabetes, and degenerative diseases. Figs are also a good source of vitamins B1, B3, B5, B9, as well as minerals iron, magnesium, potassium, and copper.

Research studies suggest that chlorogenic acid in figs help lower blood sugar levels and control blood-glucose levels in type 2 diabetes.

Garlic

Garlic is perhaps best known for its antibacterial, antifungal properties. It is loaded with minerals such as copper, potassium, calcium, manganese, zinc, iron, magnesium, and phosphorus. Garlic is also rich in protein and vitamins B1, B2, and C. Garlic is a great natural remedy for getting rid of common colds.

Ginger Root

Ginger is loaded with vitamins C and E, copper, potassium, calcium, manganese, iron, and magnesium. Researchers believe that ginger thins the blood and has similar effects on blood clots as aspirin. It reduces inflammation in the body, lowers high cholesterol, knocks out fevers, migraines, dizziness, and nausea. Ginger possesses therapeutic antioxidant effects and direct anti-inflammatory effects, especially for painful arthritis. Ginger is very effective in preventing motion sickness, and it promotes the elimination of intestinal gas.

Grape Leaves

Grape leaves are edible and they are good for you. The most powerful healing properties of grape leaves come from resveratrol, which has been found to act as an antioxidant, antimutagen, and anti-inflammatory. Resveratrol has also been shown to inhibit the development of breast cancer and myelocytic leukemia. According to herbalist and nutritionist Donald Yance, grape leaves are the best source of resveratrol—they are up to one hundred times richer in resveratrol than the grapes. An anti-inflammatory, resveratrol increases energy levels, lowers blood sugar, and extends life.

Grape leaves are an excellent source of vitamin A. They are a good source of many other nutrients, including vitamins C, E, K, B3, and B6, plus iron, fiber, riboflavin, folate, calcium, potassium, magnesium, copper, phosphorus, choline, and manganese.

Fresh grape leaves contain about 3 percent fat, an unexpectedly large amount for a green, most of which is omega-3.

Eating grape leaves can reduce edema, or fluid retention, in people with chronic venous insufficiency. Studies found that patients who received grape leaf extract showed improved microvascular blood flow, which can help prevent conditions such as varicose veins, spider veins, or chronic leg swelling.

Grape leaves may also protect the skin from sunburn and sun-induced skin aging. Resveratrol activates anti-aging genes in grape leaves that are known to protect the brain from memory loss, possibly aiding in Alzheimer's prevention.

Red grape leaves have been traditionally used to treat diarrhea, inflammation, hemorrhoids, heavy menstrual bleeding, and uterine hemorrhage.

Grapefruit

Grapefruit is an excellent source of vitamin C and is rich in phytonutrients such as vitamin A, beta-carotene, and lycopene. Just one-half of a grapefruit provides 80 percent of your recommended dietary allowance of vitamin C and 6 percent of vitamin A. Vitamin C is a powerful natural antioxidant and helps the body develop resistance against infectious agents and scavenge harmful free radicals. Vitamin A helps to protect from lung and oral-cavity cancers.

Grapefruit also contains several other vitamins—E, B2, B6, and B9—as well as minerals, including calcium, manganese, magnesium, phosphorus, and potassium.

Grapefruit consists of only 42 calories per 100 grams. However, it is rich in the dietary insoluble fiber pectin, which helps to protect the colon mucous membrane by working as a laxative, as well as binding to cancer-causing chemicals in the colon. Pectin can also reduce blood cholesterol levels by decreasing re-absorption of cholesterol-binding bile acids in the colon.

Grapes

Grapes are a great source of vitamins A, B1, B2, B6, and C. They are also rich in flavonoids, phenolic acids, and resveratrol, all of which are invaluable phytonutrients known as polyphenols. These compounds appear to decrease the risk of heart disease.

Grapes have many health benefits. The hydrating power of grapes is high, which increases the moisture present in the lungs and reduces asthmatic events. Grapes give a healthy boost to your immune system, and help with acne and other skin problems.

Grapes also help cleanse the liver and kidneys, and they even help fight night blindness.

Red grape skins and seeds contain recently isolated compounds called procyanidin B dimers that have been shown to reduce the size of estrogen-dependent breast cancer tumors.

Green Onions

Green onions are rich in chromium, vitamin C, fiber, manganese, vitamin B6, tryptophan, folate, potassium, phosphorus, and copper. Green onions lower blood sugar, decrease the risk of high cholesterol and high blood pressure, reduce the risk of colon cancer, and help rid the body of inflammation.

Guavas

Guavas are low in saturated fat, cholesterol, and sodium. They are also high in dietary fiber, vitamins C and A, folate, potassium, copper, and manganese. Guavas strengthen and tone the digestive system and can help cure dysentery by inhibiting microbial growth and removing extra mucus from the intestines. Guavas have been found to be beneficial for people suffering a number of physical ailments, including acidosis, asthma, bacterial infections, catarrh, congestion of the lungs, convulsions, epilepsy, high blood pressure, obesity, oral ulcers, poor circulation, prolonged menstruation, scurvy, and swollen gums.

Honey

Raw honey, which has not been pasteurized or filtered, is full of superb nutritional values and medicinal remedies. Honey is a source of carbohydrates, containing 80 percent natural sugar, fructose, and glucose.

The vitamins present in honey are B1, B2, B3, B5, and B6. The minerals found in honey include calcium, copper, iron, magnesium, manganese, phosphorus, potassium, sodium, and zinc.

Raw honey also contains antioxidants, present in the form of polyphenols, which help fight off free radicals that contribute to many serious diseases.

Honey is helpful against allergies and hay fever, and one or two teaspoons last thing at night can help with insomnia. Honey is effective over burns. It cools, removes pain, and helps fast healing without scarring. It contains antibiotic and anti-bacterial properties. A teaspoon of honey before bed aids water retention and helps in prevention of bed-wetting.

Similar to bee pollen, honey is the food of young bees and as such strict vegans may choose to exclude it from their diets; for this reason in our recipes we say "optional" in parentheses.

Honeydew

An excellent source of vitamin C, honeydew melon is a very good source of potassium, copper, and B vitamins, including B1, B3, B5, and B6. Honeydew is a great source of folate, which has recently been found to prevent birth defects. Folate is an essential component when cells are dividing rapidly, because it carries fragments of proteins. Honeydew melons contain plenty of water, which can keep you hydrated on a hot summer day.

Horseradish

Horseradish is laden with B vitamins, vitamin C, potassium, calcium, iron, sodium, and natural antibiotics. Due to its antibiotic properties, horseradish can cure urinary-tract infections and kill bacteria in the throat that cause bronchitis and coughs. Horseradish stimulates appetite, has aphrodisiac properties, and can cure toothaches.

Horsetail

Horsetail is a wild edible plant, rich in silicic acid, palustrine, palustridine, phytosterol, beta-sitosterol, malic acid, vitamin C, volatile oil, potassium, and natural salts. The active components in horsetail have antimicrobial, antiseptic, and anti-inflammatory effects. They preserve eyesight and stimulate blood flow. Horsetail is used to treat hyperacidity, bladder problems, dandruff, bleeding gums, and stomach and intestinal ailments.

Jackfruit

Jackfruit is an excellent source of vitamin A, which has powerful antioxidant properties and is essential for vision. It is a good source of vitamin C, a powerful antioxidant. Jackfruit is made of soft, easily digestible flesh (bulbs) with simple sugars like fructose and sucrose. Jackfruit is also rich in antioxidant flavonoids like beta-carotene and lutein. These antioxidants are found to protect against colon, prostate, breast, endometrial, lung, and pancreatic cancers. Jackfruit is rich in B-complex vitamins. It contains very good amounts of vitamins B6, B3, B2, and folate. Jackfruit is a good source of magnesium, manganese, iron, and potassium, an important component of cell and body fluids that helps control heart rate and blood pressure.

Kale

Kale is well known for its anti-inflammatory properties. High in beta-carotene, vitamins K and C, lutein, zeaxanthin, and calcium, kale contains sulforaphane, a chemical that has potent anticancer properties. Kale is also a source of indole-3-carbinol, a chemical that boosts DNA repair in cells and appears to block the growth of cancer cells.

Kelp

Kelp is an excellent source of iodine and vitamin K, a very good source of folate and magnesium, and a good source of iron, calcium, B2, and B5. Kelp also contains measurable amounts of vitamins C and E. Increased iodine intake can provide important health benefits for people with hypothyroidism. The vanadium content of kelp may help increase cells' sensitivity to insulin, help prevent overproduction of glucose by cells, thereby helping to increase blood sugar control and lower the risk of type 2 diabetes.

Kiwis

One kiwi has more than 120 percent of the recommended daily allowance of vitamin C. Besides helping to boost the immune system, vitamin C is an antioxidant that can protect arteries from the damaging effects of free radicals. Kiwi fruits are also rich in dietary fiber and are another great source of potassium, copper, magnesium, vitamin E, and manganese.

Kombucha

Kombucha tea is made from the fermentation of a mixture of sweetened tea and scoby, which is a symbiotic colony of bacteria and yeast. Kombucha has been researched in several countries, including China, Russia, and Germany. General conclusions were that kombucha contains strong antibacterial, antibiotic, and detoxifying properties and its high content of glucaric acid can aid in the prevention and treatment of cancer.

Günther Frank, in his book *Kombucha—Healthy Beverage and Natural Remedy from the Far East,* published in 1989, tells several stories associated with successful treatments of cancer. Among other stories, Frank described how the Nobel Prize–winning Russian author Aleksandr Solzhenitsyn wrote in his autobiography that his stomach cancer was cured by the regular consumption of kombucha tea. After President Ronald Reagan came to know about the author's claim, he decided to use kombucha tea to prevent his own cancer from spreading. The president survived his cancer, and he died of old age in 2004.

Kombucha tea is very rich in antioxidants, which can suppress the activities of free radicals that can cause serious damage to your body. It is also rich in B vitamins and probiotic bacteria that help to heal your gut and build your immunity.

Lamb's-quarters

Lamb's-quarters are loaded with protein, vitamins A, C, B1, B2, and B3, and essential minerals like iron, calcium, phosphorus, and potassium. Like all dark greens, lamb's-quarters fight and prevent cancer, help with diabetes, reduce inflammation, and strengthen bones.

Lemons

Lemons are jam-packed with vitamin C, one of the most important antioxidants in nature. Vitamin C travels through the body, neutralizing any free radicals it encounters. Free radicals can damage healthy cells, causing inflammation, or painful swelling, in the body. Vitamin C has been shown to be helpful for reducing some of the symptoms of osteoarthritis and rheumatoid arthritis. Antioxidants fight free radicals and help prevent cancer. Vitamin C is also vital to the function of a strong immune system. The immune system's main goal is to protect the body from illness, so a little extra vitamin C may be useful with conditions like colds, flu, and recurrent ear infections. Research has shown that daily consumption of vitamin C is associated with a reduced risk of death from all causes, including heart disease, stroke, and cancer.

Lemons also contain a variety of phytochemicals. Hesperetin and naringenin are flavonoid glycosides commonly found in citrus fruits. Naringenin is found to have a bioactive effect on human health as an antioxidant, free-radical scavenger, anti-inflammatory, and immune-system modulator. Naringenin has also been shown to reduce oxidant injury to DNA in the cells. In addition, lemons contain a healthy amount of minerals like iron, copper, potassium, and calcium. Potassium is an important component of cell and body fluids and helps control heart rate and blood pressure.

Lettuce

All lettuce is known to help with acid indigestion, anemia, arthritis, catarrh, circulatory problems, colitis, constipation, cough, diabetes, gastritis, gout, insomnia, irritable bowel, obesity, stress, tuberculosis, ulcers, and urinary-tract diseases.

Butter Head Lettuce

Butter head lettuce is tender and has mildly flavored leaves.

Butter leaf lettuce is a good source of vitamins K and C, as well as vitamin A, which is beneficial for skin, eyes, and mucus membranes such as the lips. Butter head lettuce also contains a great amount of fiber, folate, calcium, iron, potassium, and bioflavonoids. It is also a good source of phytonutrients, organic compounds that fight against disease. One of these phytonutrients is carotenoid zeaxanthin. When consumed, zeaxanthin is absorbed into the retinal macula in the eye. There, it acts as an antioxidant and helps protect the eye from harmful light.

Green Leaf Lettuce

Green leaf lettuce contains large amounts of vitamins A and K, plus the antioxidants beta-carotene and lutein, which are beneficial for weak eyes.

Miner's Lettuce

Miner's lettuce is loaded with vitamins A and C. It was traditionally used by early pioneers to combat scurvy and heart conditions caused by lack of vitamin C.

Red Leaf Lettuce

Red leaf lettuce has the most vitamin A, vitamin B6, and antioxidants of all the lettuces. Red leaf lettuce is beneficial for weak eyes, helps to repair blood vessels, and has an anticancer effect.

Romaine Lettuce

Romaine is rich in antioxidants, which are believed to help prevent cancer, and is beneficial in the treatment of insomnia, as it contains a sleep-inducing substance. Romaine is an excellent source of vitamin A, folate, vitamin C, manganese, and chromium. In addition, romaine is a very good source of dietary fiber, vitamins B1 and B2, and the minerals potassium, molybdenum, iron, and phosphorus.

Limes

Limes have similar nutritional and health benefits to lemons. An excellent source of vitamin C, limes offer good amounts of folate, vitamin B6, potassium, flavonoids, and the important phytochemical limonene. Limes contain phytochemicals that are high in antioxidant and anticancer properties. Studies have shown that lime juice can affect cell cycles, stopping cell division in many cancer cell lines or boosting the activity of white blood cells. Limes also have an antibiotic effect and strongly protect against diseases such as cholera.

Mallow (Malva)

Mallow is a good source of calcium, magnesium, potassium, iron, selenium, and vitamins A and C. Mallow has been found to be beneficial for many different conditions, including Crohn's disease, asthma, gastritis, indigestion, and ulcerative colitis.

Mangos

Mangos are rich in vitamins C and A. They also have traces of vitamins E, B6, and K and the mineral selenium. Mangos contain phenols, chemical compounds with powerful antioxidant and anticancer abilities. Mangos are also rich in iron, which makes them great for pregnant women and people with anemia. The nutritional value of mangos makes them beneficial for weight gain, eye disorders, hair loss, heat stroke, prickly heat, diabetes, bacterial infections, sinusitis, piles, indigestion, constipation, morning sickness, diarrhea, dysentery, scurvy, spleen enlargement, liver disorders, menstrual disorders, leucorrhoea, and vaginitis.

Mint

Any fresh mint (spearmint, peppermint, etc.) is rich in vitamins A, C, B1, and B2 and folate, as well as the essential minerals manganese, magnesium, copper, potassium, iron, calcium, zinc, phosphorus, fluoride, and selenium. All mints help soothe the stomach and aid the digestive tract. Mint has been used to treat upset stomach, nausea, morning sickness, and irritable bowel syndrome. Mint also has anticancer properties.

Mizuna Greens

Mizuna (pronounced "meezuna") is one of the mildest-tasting mustard greens, often available during cold seasons.

Mizuna is high in immune-boosting vitamin C, which enhances the immune system, and is high in vitamin E, folate, calcium, potassium, chromium, selenium, molybdenum, and iron.

Mizuna greens contain powerful antioxidants known as glucosinolates that have the capability to reduce the risk of acquiring cancer.

Mulberries

Mulberries contain more protein than perhaps any other berry commonly found in North America. They are also a good source of calcium and phosphorus. Mulberries promote proper body fluid production and thus can balance internal secretions and enhance immunity. Mulberries also soothe nerves, strengthen kidneys and liver, lower cholesterol, lower hypertension, and reduce blood-sugar levels. Regular consumption of mulberries has been linked to positive changes in eyesight. In addition, it has been said that persons with graying hair can benefit from a regular intake of fresh mulberries. Mulberry juice applied directly to hair also promotes its healthy growth.

Mustard Greens

Revered throughout history as the healthiest greens, mustard greens are low in calories and contain a large number of antioxidants. They provide an excellent source of vitamins B1, B2, and B6 as well as C and E. They are also a good source of folate, calcium, beta-carotene, manganese, copper, fiber, phosphorus, magnesium, protein, potassium, and iron. Mustard greens are also especially beneficial for women who are going through menopause, because they have the ability to protect against breast cancer and heart disease. Their high nutrient content also supports bone health.

Nectarines

Nectarines are a good source of vitamin A, potassium, and soluble fiber, which help fight cancer and keep digestion running smoothly. Nectarines are also a good source of lycopene and lutein, phytochemicals that help prevent heart disease, macular degeneration, and cancer.

Nori

Among seaweeds, nori has the most nutrition. It contains as much protein as soybeans as well as twelve kinds of vitamins, including A and B-complex vitamins. You can consume enough vitamin A per day with just two sheets of nori. Two sheets of nori provide: the daily requirement of vitamin A; vitamins B1 and B2 in amounts equivalent to 50–60 grams of pork; twice the vitamin C as the same number of tangerines; and an amount of iron equal to 20 ounces of milk or one egg. Nori is a rich source of calcium, zinc, and iodine and also a good source of lignans, which help fight cancer. Nori is full of dietary fiber, which is necessary for maintaining good health.

Nutmeg

Nutmeg is rich in potassium, calcium, phosphorus, and magnesium. It has a good amount of vitamins A and C, choline, and sodium and a small amount of vitamins B1, B2, B3, B6, folate, iron, zinc, copper, manganese, and selenium. Nutmeg can relieve stomachache and diarrhea and helps to detoxify the body, reduce blood pressure, and increase blood circulation. It is also good for digestion, reducing acidity, and relieving vomiting and flatulence and is often used as a medicine for respiratory problems.

Nutritional Yeast

Nutritional yeast is an excellent source of protein (52 percent of our daily recommended allowances) containing essential amino acids. It is rich in vitamins, especially the B-complex vitamins, and is an excellent source of folate, which is important for the formation of red blood cells.

Olive Oil

Olive oil is rich in monounsaturated fat and antioxidants like chlorophyll, carotenoids, and vitamin E. Scientists have identified a compound in olive oil, called oleuropein, that prevents the LDL cholesterol from oxidizing. Replacing other fats in your diet with olive oil can significantly lower blood pressure and reduce the risk of heart attack. Olive oil has been shown to reduce the effect of oncogenes, which are associated with the rapid growth of breast-cancer tumors. Researchers discovered that the oleic acid in olive oil encouraged the self-destruction of cancer cells. Olive oil has been positively indicated in studies on prostate and endometrial cancers as well.

Oranges

Oranges are an excellent source vitamin C, a powerful antioxidant that neutralizes harmful elements within the body. Vitamin C also stimulates the absorption of nonheme iron, thus reducing iron deficiency, and keeps the immune system strong and healthy. Vitamin C also helps maintain collagen, the substance that helps the human body repair tissue.

Oranges are high in fiber. A single orange provides 12.5 percent of the daily value for fiber, which has been shown to reduce high cholesterol and atherosclerosis. The high fiber content in oranges can help keep blood-sugar levels from rising too high after eating. Studies show that food rich in fiber may provide a line of protection from colon cancer. Fiber from oranges can also reduce constipation or diarrhea in those suffering from irritable bowel syndrome. In addition, oranges are a good source of vitamin B1, folate, vitamin A (in the form of beta-carotene), potassium, and calcium.

Oregano

Oregano has been shown to provide forty-two times more antioxidant activity than apples. As a matter of fact, ounce for ounce, oregano is thought to be one of the most antioxidant-dense foods. Oregano is known to have strong antibacterial properties, as its powerful essential oils inhibit the growth of many kinds of bacteria, including some that cause serious food-borne illnesses. Oregano is a very good source of iron, manganese, and dietary fiber as well as calcium, vitamins C and A, and omega-3 fatty acids. Vitamins A and C are powerful antioxidants, which play a vital role in the prevention of many forms of cancer as well as in slowing down the aging process.

Papayas

Papayas are a rich source of antioxidant nutrients, including carotenes, vitamin C, and flavonoids; the vitamins B6 and B9; the minerals potassium and magnesium; and fiber. Together, these nutrients promote the health of the cardiovascular system and provide protection against colon cancer. In addition, papain, an enzyme found in papayas, is used to treat sports injuries, other causes of trauma, and allergies. Papayas also contain the important enzyme arginine, which is known to be essential for male fertility. Papayas are also a good source of fiber, which has been shown to lower high cholesterol levels.

Parsley

Parsley contains large amounts of vitamins A, C, and E as well as iron, manganese, calcium, and potassium. The vitamin C is not only useful in its own right, but also assists in the absorption of iron. Parsley is beneficial against kidney stones and rheumatism and for settling the stomach and improving appetite. Parsley's volatile oils—particularly myristicin—have been shown to inhibit tumor formation. Owing to the high quantity of vitamin A (for beauty) and vitamin E (for elasticity) in parsley, it can also be used for cosmetic purposes, specifically as a restorative face tonic.

Peaches

Peaches have vitamins A, C, B1, B2, and B3, fiber, iron, calcium, potassium, magnesium, and phosphorus. Peaches have been noted to make skin healthy and add color to complexion. The consumption of peaches helps remove worms and other parasites from the intestinal tract. Peaches are also high in antioxidants, and their flowers have been found to have mild sedative properties, which make them a great organic option for people suffering from insomnia.

Pears, Asian Pears

Pears are a great source of fiber, vitamins B2, C, and E as well as copper and potassium. They are also an excellent source of pectin, a water-soluble fiber, which makes them a great natural remedy for high cholesterol. A hypoallergenic fruit, pears are less likely to produce an adverse allergic response. Perhaps for this reason, pears are often recommended as a safe fruit to introduce to infants.

Peas

Green peas provide nutrients that are important for maintaining bone health. They are a very good source of vitamin K, folate, and vitamin B6. The latter two nutrients help to reduce the buildup of a metabolic by-product called homocysteine, a dangerous molecule that can obstruct collagen cross-linking, which results in poor bone density and osteoporosis. They also support cardiovascular health. Green peas are a very good source of vitamins B1, B2, and B3, all of which are necessary for metabolism. Green peas are also a good source of iron, a mineral necessary for normal blood-cell formation and function, whose deficiency results in anemia, fatigue, decreased immune function, and learning problems. Green peas are a very good source of vitamin C, which protects many energy-producing cells and systems in the body from free-radical damage. Body tissues with particularly high vitamin C requirements include the adrenal glands, ocular lens, liver, immune system, and connective tissues. Vitamin C is instrumental in helping to prevent the development of cancer.

Peppers

Jalapeño Peppers

Jalapeños are a good source of vitamin C, folate, and vitamin A. Capsaicin, the chemical that makes chili peppers hot, is capable of killing off cancer cells without damaging healthy cells. Studies show that chili peppers can provide pain relief for migraine and sinus headaches. Heat from jalapeños helps stimulate secretions that aid in clearing mucus from the chest and nose, effectively combating nasal congestion. Jalapeños also have antibacterial properties that help fight chronic sinus infections. If consumed thirty minutes prior to exercise, chili peppers can double the amount of fat burned during a workout.

Red Bell Peppers

Bell peppers also contain a large number of phytochemicals that have exceptional antioxidant capabilities. These antioxidants work together to effectively neutralize free radicals, which can travel through the body and cause damage to cells. By providing these potent free-radical destroyers, bell peppers may help prevent or reduce some of the following symptoms: cholesterol in the arteries that leads to atherosclerosis and heart disease, the nerve and blood-vessel damage seen in diabetes, the cloudy lenses of cataracts, the joint pain and damage seen in osteoarthritis and rheumatoid arthritis, and the wheezing and airway tightening of asthma.

Red peppers contain lycopene, a carotenoid whose consumption has been correlated with protection against prostate cancer and cancers of the cervix, bladder, and pancreas. Red bell peppers contain lutein and zeaxanthin, the phytonutrients that have been found to protect against macular degeneration, the main cause of blindness in the elderly. Other phytochemicals in red bell peppers include chlorogenic acid and coumaric acid. Studies have shown that red bell peppers have significantly higher levels of nutrients than other varieties.

Yellow Bell Peppers

Yellow bell peppers are loaded with vitamins C and A, two very powerful antioxidants that have been shown to prevent blood clots and reduce the risk of heart attacks and strokes. Bell peppers also contain vitamins B1 and B6 and folate. Phytochemicals include chlorogenic acid, zeaxanthin, and coumaric acid.

Persimmons

Persimmons are high in calcium, iron, phosphorus, and vitamins C and A. The fruit is low in calories (provides 70 calories/100g) and fats but is a rich source of dietary fiber.

Persimmons have been used in traditional Chinese medicine to remedy hiccups. They have also been used to treat diarrhea, hemorrhoids, lung infections, and asthma.

Pineapple

Pineapple is an excellent source of vitamin C and the trace mineral manganese, an essential cofactor in a number of enzymes important in energy production and antioxidant defenses. Just one cup of fresh pineapple supplies 128 percent of the daily recommended amount of manganese. In addition to manganese, pineapple is a good source of vitamin B1, which acts as a cofactor in enzymatic reactions central to energy production. Regular consumption of pineapple has been linked to regulating and preventing goiters and the enlargement of the thyroid gland. Pineapples are also associated with benefits such as regulating blood pressure and combating arthritis, intestinal worms, constipation, and throat infections. One of the most important enzymes in pineapple is bromelain, which has been found to have anti-inflammatory properties, thus helping to reduce swelling and assisting in the treatment of conditions such as acute sinusitis, sore throat, arthritis, and gout.

Plantain

In this book we talk about plantain that is a common weed (not a banana). Its Latin name is *Plantago major* ("broadleaf plantain" or "greater plantain").

The leaves of plantain contain calcium and other minerals, with 100 grams of plantain containing approximately the same amount of vitamin A as a large carrot.

Plantain is very rich in tannin, which helps draw tissues together to stop bleeding. It also contains allantoin, a compound that promotes healing of injured skin cells. Further studies have indicated that plantain may also reduce blood pressure.

Plantain is effective in treating obesity, as it has an appetite-satiating effect and reduces intestinal absorption of liquids. Plantain is highly antiseptic, anti-inflammatory, antifungal, and antiviral. It speeds up wound healing and stops bleeding and itching; direct leaf contact immediately improves physical injuries, insect bites, and poison ivy. It also works great on eczema, dandruff, sunburn, and diaper rash. In Europe plantain is used as a cough, cold, and bronchitis remedy.

When used in salads, plantain is known as a digestive aid. Plantain has been used as a remedy for many other conditions, such as indigestion, constipation, diarrhea, dysentery, uterine toner, anti-cancerous (slows and represses tumor growth), anti-cardiovascular disease (as it lowers LDL cholesterol and improves HDL and also lowers triglycerides), eye wash, epilepsy, tuberculosis, gastric and bowel ulcers, and dyspepsia.

Plums

Plums are a good source of health-promoting flavonoid polyphenolic antioxidants such as lutein, cryptoxanthin, and zeaxanthin in significant amounts. These compounds help act as scavengers against oxygen-derived free radicals and reactive oxygen species (ROS) that play a role in aging and various disease processes. In addition, plums are rich in potassium, fiber, and vitamin C and have elements that are beneficial to eyesight.

Pomegranate Seeds

Pomegranates are rich in punicalagins, a potent antioxidant responsible for pomegranates' superior health benefits. The antioxidant level is even higher in pomegranates than in blueberries, cranberries, and oranges, largely because of pomegranates' high level of polyphenols; they thus help support the body's normal defense in the prevention of certain cancers and keep LDL cholesterol from oxidizing, which can lead to atherosclerosis.

Pomegranates are also a good source of vitamins B1, B2, B3, and C, calcium, and phosphorus, all of which prevent and reverse many diseases. Pomegranates may reduce the risk of heart disease, heart attacks, and strokes and are rumored to help reduce the possibility of having premature babies and Alzheimer's disease. In addition, pomegranate juice, like aspirin, can help keep blood platelets from clumping together to form unwanted clots. Some researchers report that long-term consumption of pomegranate juice may help combat erectile dysfunction. Investigators are also excited about the possibility that pomegranate compounds might prevent prostate cancer or slow its growth.

Prickly Pears

Prickly pear is a cactus fruit that is a good source of vitamin C, calcium, magnesium, and copper and an excellent source of fiber, which helps the digestive system. Prickly pears can reduce brain swelling and are often used for hangover cures. These cactus fruits have been revered for stabilizing blood-sugar levels and are thus good for diabetics. Prickly pears also alleviate sore muscles, cleanse the colon, and have been used as an effective aid in weight loss. Prickly pears' amino acids have been associated with the benefit of lowering high cholesterol and cleaning up the arteries, which reduces the formation of plaque while improving circulation.

Prunes

Prunes are a good source of vitamin A and other antioxidants, which help to eliminate free radicals that would otherwise cause a lot of damage to cells and cell membranes. Prunes are a good source of potassium and increase absorption of iron into the body. They promote normal blood circulation, slow the aging process, help anemia, and contain sorbitol, a stool-softening agent, which helps prevent constipation.

Psyllium

Psyllium is the husk of the seed of the plantain plant, which is a common wild edible.

Psyllium husk powder provides the much-needed dietary fiber to those who consume fiber-deficient diets. Every 100 grams of psyllium provides 71 grams of soluble fiber. For comparison, 100 grams of oat bran would contain only 5 grams of soluble fiber. Psyllium husk powder is the strongest natural dietary fiber for promoting regularity and supporting heart health as well as for promotion of digestive regularity.

Psyllium husk powder helps your body maintain healthy blood-sugar levels as it works in your digestive system by gelling and trapping sugars so they can be slowly released and absorbed in your body.

Pumpkin Leaves

Pumpkin leaves are a great source of vitamins C and B6, folate, calcium, iron, magnesium, phosphorus, potassium, copper, manganese, protein, and omega-3 fatty acids. Dark green pumpkin leaves contain a large amount of vitamin A, which is vital for proper growth, healthy eyes, and strong immunity.

Purslane (Portulaca)

Purslane contains more omega-3 fatty acids than some fish oils. Research shows that consumption of foods rich in omega-3 fatty acids may reduce the risk of coronary heart disease and stroke and also help prevent the development of ADHD, autism, and developmental problems in children. Purslane's vitamin A content is one of the highest among green leafy vegetables (100 grams yield 44 percent of the recommended daily allowance). Vitamin A, a known powerful natural antioxidant, is essential for vision and for healthy mucus membranes and skin. The consumption of natural vegetables and fruits rich in vitamin A has been known to help protect from lung and oral-cavity cancers. Purslane is also a rich source of vitamin C, some B vitamins (B2, B3, B6), and carotenoids as well as dietary minerals such as iron, magnesium, calcium, potassium, and manganese.

Raspberries

Raspberries are an excellent source of manganese and vitamin C, two critical antioxidant nutrients that help protect the body's cells from oxygen-related damage. Raspberries are also a good source of vitamins B2 and B3, folate, magnesium, potassium, and copper. This fruit is packed with fiber and manganese, both of which help keep your metabolic rate high, which in turn burns fat. Fiber helps slow the digestive process so you feel full longer. This combination of nutrients makes raspberries a great fruit choice for having minimal impact on blood sugars. Research has suggested that raspberries have the potential to inhibit cancer-cell proliferation and tumor formation in various parts of the body, including the colon.

Rosemary

Rosemary promotes circulation and thus can improve health problems such as Alzheimer's disease, eczema, rheumatic disorders, and yeast infections. It is rich in vitamins A, C, and others, along with minerals with antioxidant, antiseptic, antispasmodic, diuretic, and fungicidal properties. The substances contained in rosemary are useful for stimulating the immune system, increasing circulation, and improving digestion. Rosemary also contains anti-inflammatory compounds that may make it useful for reducing the severity of asthma attacks. In addition, rosemary has been shown to increase blood flow to the head and brain, improving concentration.

Sage

Sage is an herb with a pleasant aroma. Sage is often used as a fragrance in soaps and cosmetics.

Sage contains very good amounts of vitamins A, C, and K. Sage leaves are a rich source of minerals like potassium, zinc, calcium, iron, manganese, copper, and magnesium. Potassium helps control heart rate and blood pressure.

Sage is used in medicine to help alleviate symptoms of digestive problems and mental disorders, such as Alzheimer's and depression.

Sauerkraut

Sauerkraut has multiple health benefits, including providing fiber and a significant amount of vitamins C and K. Sauerkraut enhances your digestive system with a diverse population of live bacteria. These probiotics replenish the good bacteria in your gut and help inhibit the growth of bad bacteria. They may also boost your immune system and synthesize B vitamins.

Sorrel

Sorrel is an excellent source of three vitamins: C, A, and folate. A good source of magnesium and calcium, sorrel is also high in iron, which makes sorrel beneficial for hepatitis, liver disorders, constipation, blood disorders, skin disease, rheumatism, rashes, and insect bites and stings. It can also help remove heavy metals from the body.

Spinach

Spinach is extremely rich in antioxidants vitamins A (and especially high in lutein), C, and E; vitamins B2, B3, B6, K, folate, and betaine; protein; iron, magnesium, manganese, calcium, potassium, copper, phosphorus, zinc, and selenium; and omega-3 fatty acids. Due to substances like choline and inositol, which are present in significant amounts, spinach helps the arteries remain healthy.

Diabetics can particularly benefit from spinach, which is known to stabilize blood sugar and prevent fluctuations. Flavonoids and carotenoids present in spinach are powerful antioxidants and have anticancer effects. Spinach is known to be an anti-aging vegetable and, rich in vitamin K, spinach helps in the clotting of blood in case of injuries.

Sprouts

Sprouts are loaded with highly active antioxidants that prevent DNA destruction and protect from the ongoing effects of aging. All sprouts are rich in plant estrogens, which increase bone formation and density and prevent osteoporosis. They are also helpful in controlling hot flashes, menopause, PMS, and fibrocystic breast tumors.

Alfalfa Sprouts

Alfalfa sprouts contain canavanine, an amino-acid analog that is beneficial against pancreatic, colon, and leukemia cancers. Regular consumption of alfalfa sprouts provides benefits against arteriosclerosis and cardiovascular disease. Alfalfa sprouts are rich in saponins, which lower the bad cholesterol (LDL), but not the good (HDL). Saponins also stimulate the immune system by increasing the activity of natural killer cells such as T- lymphocytes and interferons. The saponin content of alfalfa sprouts is 450 percent greater than that in the unsprouted seed.

Broccoli Sprouts

Multiple researchers concluded that broccoli sprouts promoted much more (twenty to fifty times more) cancer protection and antioxidant activity than broccoli alone.

Buckwheat Sprouts

Buckwheat sprouts are high in iron, so they are a good blood builder. They also prevent osteoporosis because of their high boron and calcium levels. Sprouted buckwheat is high in flavonoids and co-enzyme Q10. It contains all of the B vitamins, tryptophan, magnesium, manganese, and selenium, as well as many other health-giving compounds.

Buckwheat sprouts help relax blood vessels and improve blood flow, which is beneficial for people who have varicose veins or hardening of the arteries. One of the reasons is that they are full of rutin, which is a powerful capillary-wall strengthener. The high level of magnesium in buckwheat sprouts has been shown to lower the risk of diabetes. The high plant-lignan content in buckwheat sprouts helps prevent heart disease and some cancers.

Sunflower Sprouts

Sunflower greens provide a well-balanced form of a complete plant protein, which helps to repair muscle tissue.

Sunflower greens are an excellent source of vitamins C, E, A, D, and E, as well as folate, a vital nutrient for pregnant women and developing babies.

Sunflower greens are a good source of important minerals, including calcium, copper, iron, phosphorous, magnesium, selenium, and potassium.

Vitamin D in sunflower sprouts builds strong bones and muscles and is associated with controlling blood pressure. Sunflower sprouts are also a good source of lecithin, a phospholipid compound that aids in the body's transport of fats.

Star Fruit

Star fruit are very rich in vitamins A and C as well as potassium, phosphorous, iron, and calcium. They are also a good source of fiber, amino acids, and antioxidants. Besides the known benefits of their vitamin and mineral composition for skin health, nerve functions, healthy bones, digestion, blood oxygenation, and cancer prevention, star fruit are also known to be effective in hormone regulation, specifically in the thyroid gland, as well as in regulating appetite and sleep, making it helpful in the diets of families with small children. It is also a popular home remedy in treating fevers, headaches, and even hangovers.

Stinging Nettles

A cup of stinging nettles contains 1,790 IU of vitamin A, nearly three times the amount you need in a single day. Stinging nettles also provide an excellent source of vitamin K, a vitamin your body requires for blood clotting.

Stinging nettles are an excellent source of potassium, calcium, magnesium, manganese, phosphorous, and iron, which is important to combat anemia or attention-deficit hyperactivity disorder.

For over two thousand years, doctors have recognized stinging nettles' ability to stop all kinds of internal and external bleeding, and have considered it a good blood purifier. Nettle has been used for centuries to treat allergy symptoms, particularly hay fever, which is the most common allergy problem.

Nettle has been studied extensively and has shown promise in treating Alzheimer's disease, arthritis, asthma, bladder infections, edema, bronchitis, bursitis, gingivitis, gout, hives, kidney stones, laryngitis, multiple sclerosis, PMS, prostate enlargement, sciatica, and tendinitis! Nettle may lower blood pressure and heart rate. It may also lower blood sugar.

Strawberries

Strawberries are an excellent source of vitamins C and K, fiber, and flavonoids. They are also a very good source of vitamins B1 and B5, iodine, and manganese and a good source of vitamin B6, folate, and biotin. Strawberries have been linked with numerous health benefits, such as reducing ocular pressure, promoting proper eyesight, and fighting cancer, arthritis, gout, and high blood pressure. Regular consumption of strawberries has also been said to promote proper brain function.

Sweet Potato Leaves

Sweet potato leaves are a by-product of the plant and a good source of nutrients. They are high in fiber, beta-carotene, lutein, vitamin K, and folate. They are also high in minerals: potassium, phosphorus, magnesium, sodium, manganese, zinc, and copper. All of these nutrients help reduce inflammation and fight diseases, such as diabetes, heart ailments, hypertension, and various forms of cancer.

Sweet potato leaves are also rich in vitamins C and E, which help to fight off free radicals and boost the immune system.

Swiss Chard

Swiss chard is high in fiber, protein, vitamins A, C, E, K, B1, B2, B6, calcium, tryptophan, iron, magnesium, phosphorus, potassium, copper, manganese, sodium, folate, and zinc. Swiss chard is ideal for weight loss and maintaining optimum health. Swiss chard is a unique source of phytonutrients called betalains, which provide antioxidant, anti-inflammatory, and detoxification support.

Tangerines

Tangerines contain high levels of vitamins C and A and are a very good source of fiber. They have been used as an effective remedy for breaking fevers and cleansing the liver. Tangerines have a high water content, which helps hydrate the body and keep it running smoothly.

Tatsoi Greens

Tatsoi greens have a soft creamy texture and a subtle but distinctive flavor. Tatsoi greens are loaded with calcium. One cup of fresh, chopped tatsoi greens, for example, provides almost a third of the daily value for calcium.

Tatsoi greens are very high in vitamins A, C, and K. Tatsoi also contains potassium, phosphorous, and iron and helps to strengthen the liver, blood, and bones.

Tomatillos

Tomatillos are loaded with protein, vitamins A, C, and K, iron, lycopene, potassium, flavonoids, and folate and are known to have anti-cancer properties. Tomatillos are a great choice for low-glycemic smoothies, as they have relatively low sugar content.

Tomatoes

One of the best-known benefits of tomatoes is their high lycopene content. A vital antioxidant, lycopene helps fight against cancerous cell formation as well as other kinds of health complications and diseases. Lycopene is not produced naturally within the body, so the human body requires outside sources of this powerful antioxidant. Although other fruits and vegetables do contain lycopene, no other fruit or vegetable has as high a concentration of lycopene as tomatoes do. Tomatoes are an excellent source of vitamins C and A, the latter notably through its concentration of carotenoids, including beta-carotene. These antioxidants travel through the body, neutralizing dangerous free radicals that could otherwise damage cells and cell membranes, escalating inflammation and the progression or severity of atherosclerosis, diabetic complications, asthma, and colon cancer. In fact, high intakes of these antioxidants have been shown to help reduce the risk or severity of all of these illnesses.

Tomatoes are known blood purifiers, have anti-inflammatory properties, and have been said to improve skin texture and color. They are a very good source of potassium, vitamins B3 and B6, and folate. Vitamin B3 (niacin) has been used for years as a safe way to lower high cholesterol levels. Diets rich in potassium have been shown to lower high blood pressure and reduce the risk of heart disease. Vitamin B6 and folate are both needed by the body to convert a potentially dangerous chemical called homocysteine into other, benign molecules. High levels of homocysteine, which can directly damage blood-vessel walls, are associated with an increased risk of heart attack and stroke. All of these nutrients work together to make tomatoes a truly heart-healthy food.

Turmeric

Turmeric contains the active ingredient curcumin, a powerful compound that gives turmeric its therapeutic benefits, yellow color, and pungent flavor. More specifically, curcumin has antioxidant, anti-inflammatory, antibacterial, stomach-soothing, liver- and heart-protecting effects. As an antioxidant, curcumin is helpful in many diseases, such as arthritis, where free radicals are responsible for painful joint inflammation and long-term damage to the joints. Curcumin may provide an inexpensive, well-tolerated, and effective treatment for inflammatory bowel disease (IBD), such as Crohn's disease and ulcerative colitis. According to recent studies, curcumin can correct the most common expression of the genetic defect responsible for cystic fibrosis. Curcumin also helps the body to destroy cancer cells, so they cannot spread through the body and cause more harm. A primary way in which curcumin does so is by enhancing liver function. It also inhibits cancer-cell growth and metastases. A number of studies have suggested that curcumin protects against Alzheimer's disease by turning on a gene that codes for the production of antioxidant proteins.

Turnip Greens

Turnip greens are packed with vitamins K, A, C, E, B1, B2, B3, B5, B6, folate, manganese, chromium, potassium, molybdenum, protein, tryptophan, copper, and iron. It is not surprising that with so many vitamins and minerals, turnip greens are great for combating cancer, diabetes, and inflammation. Regular consumption of turnip greens also supports digestion and heart health.

Vanilla Beans

Vanilla beans are composed of simple and complex sugars, essential oils, vitamins, and minerals. Vanilla beans contain small amounts of B-complex vitamins such as B1, B2, B3, B5, and B6. These B-complex vitamins help in enzyme synthesis, nervous system function, and regulation of the body's metabolism. Vanilla beans also contain traces of minerals such as calcium, magnesium, potassium, manganese, iron, and zinc.

Water

The human body is primarily water and needs to have its supply replenished in order to function properly. In addition to hydrating the body and preventing unnecessary cell damage, drinking water has been linked with such positive health benefits as excellent skin, relieving sore throat, aiding in weight loss, rinsing sugars off teeth, and reducing fever.

Watercress

Watercress is a rich source of minerals, including copper, calcium, potassium, magnesium, manganese, and phosphorus. Potassium is important for controlling heart rate and blood pressure by countering the effects of sodium. Manganese is used by the body as a cofactor for the antioxidant enzyme superoxide dismutase. Calcium is required for strong bones and teeth and in the regulation of heart and skeletal muscle activity. Watercress also has anticancer properties. Because watercress contains high levels of lutein and zeaxanthin, it helps protect the eyes. Watercress also increases sexual energy and enhances fertility.

Watermelon

Watermelon is loaded with powerful antioxidants, vitamins A, C, B1, and B6, potassium, magnesium, and other minerals. Watermelon is one of the most alkalizing foods. It is extremely high in water content, which helps hydrate the body. This makes watermelon a great food to consume after a strenuous workout. Watermelon is also rich in electrolytes, sodium, and potassium, all of which the body loses during perspiration. Watermelon has a special cooling effect and is exceptionally high in citrulline, an amino acid that the body uses to make another amino acid, arginine, which is used in the urea cycle to remove ammonia from the body. Watermelon is fat free, but helps energy production. It protects against macular degeneration.

Wheatgrass

Wheatgrass is one of nature's superfoods, containing vitamins, minerals, enzymes, amino acids, and large amounts of chlorophyll; it is an excellent source of calcium, iron, magnesium, phosphorus, potassium, sodium, sulfur, cobalt, and zinc.

Wheatgrass juice offers power-packed nutrition and healing properties in a concentrated and easily assimilated form, as it contains most of the vitamins and minerals needed for human maintenance. With about thirty enzymes and made up of approximately 70 percent crude chlorophyll, wheatgrass juice is an entire meal (and a complete protein). It enhances the capillaries, thereby reducing high blood pressure, improves blood formation, helps against various blood disorders, strengthens immunity, and relieves inflammation in the body. Wheatgrass juice is extremely rich in free-radical scavengers such as vitamins A and C, is believed to inhibit cancer, and improves eye health and digestion. It helps with skin problems and disorders, such as eczema and psoriasis, and is a good skin cleanser and body deodorant (it even works against graying hair). Wheatgrass juice helps to cure acne and even remove its scars, if ingested for a sustained period of eight months or so.

Zucchini

Zucchini are an excellent source of manganese and vitamin C as well as a very good source of magnesium, vitamin A, fiber, potassium, folate, copper, vitamin B2, and phosphorus. Many of these nutrients have been shown in studies to be helpful for the prevention of atherosclerosis and diabetic heart disease. Zucchini's magnesium has been shown to be helpful for reducing the risk of heart attack and stroke. Zucchini have been found to be beneficial to people suffering from asthma. Regular intake of zucchini effectively lowers high homocysteine levels in the body. Zucchini consumption can prevent multiple sclerosis.

4 Recipes for Health

Knowledge is a treasure, but practice is the key to it. —LAO TZU

People have long known that plants possess many healing properties. For this book, I looked through the particular remedial properties of different fruits, vegetables, and greens and created a compilation of recipes that may help with different conditions. The medicinal properties of plants are very mild and don't create any side effects. Of course, drinking green smoothies cannot substitute for doctor visits, but these blends might become a great aid in your healing process. Additionally, I am sure your doctors would approve of your regular consumption of greens, fruits, and veggies. The ingredients in these recipes are sold in supermarkets, health stores, and farmers' markets and are therefore easy to find.

The fact that the names of these recipes are often tied to a specific condition doesn't mean that you have to only consume the ones that strictly relate to you. Anyone can consume any of these mixes and benefit greatly from them. For example, cherries contain high levels of melatonin, which helps regulate sleeping and waking cycles. However, we all know that everybody would benefit from cherries, and particularly a person with sleep disorders. Another example is young coconut. A recent study has demonstrated that a diet rich in coconut oil protects against insulin resistance in muscle and fat, thereby helping to reverse type 2 diabetes. I have added coconut to the smoothies for diabetes, but of course anyone will become healthier by drinking such smoothies. Several recipes contain bee products, which I have marked as "optional" out of respect for vegans.

I recommend that you begin your green-smoothie journey by trying several of our blends, but don't stick to them forever; as soon as possible begin creating your own combinations. This will allow you to prepare smoothies that will best fit your personal needs and preferences. For example, some of you might enjoy the sweeter combinations, while others would choose the greener ones. Some like adding a little more water and sipping their thin smoothies, while others put in little or no water and prefer eating thick smoothies with a spoon. There are countless approaches as well as unlimited combinations, which makes green smoothies' preparation fun and adjustable to everyone's personal needs.

Please add only *ripe* fruit to your smoothies. Strive to use organically grown produce whenever possible. Remember that the main point of adding green smoothies to your diet is to benefit from their nutritional value. Blending improves two steps in the digestive process: *absorption* of nutrients into the blood and *assimilation* of nutrients from the blood into cells. Blending breaks food down into minuscule particles, which results in a much higher level of absorption and assimilation by your body.

The majority of recipes in this book have the same instructions: blend well and drink. Each recipe yields approximately two quarts of green smoothie unless otherwise stated. The recipes are grouped by topic, with topics arranged alphabetically.

Enjoy your green smoothies!

Body Boosts

Aging Gracefully

- 2 cups purslane leaves
- 1 cup red-leaf lettuce
- 2 cups fresh or frozen blackberries
- 1 cup pomegranate juice
- 1 teaspoon chia seeds
- 2 cups water

Antioxidant Blast

- 1 cup wheatgrass
- 2 cups broccoli sprouts
- 2 cups fresh or frozen blackberries
- 2 cups fresh or frozen raspberries
- Juice of ½ lemon
- ½ teaspoon turmeric
- 3 cups water

A Natural Aphrodisiac

▶ 3 stalks celery
1 cup arugula
2 sprigs basil
3 cups fresh figs
1 banana
½ teaspoon nutmeg
3 cups water

Sweet Love Cocktail

▶ 1 cup sorrel
2 cups arugula
4 cups watermelon chunks, with seeds
1 banana
1 vanilla bean
1 cup water

In-the-Mood Mix

▶ 3 stalks celery
2 cups arugula
1 banana
½ avocado, pit and skin removed
1 cup pomegranate juice
1 teaspoon cinnamon
3 cups water

Athlete's Green Power

▶ 1 cup spinach

1 cup Swiss chard, stems removed

1 cup collard greens, stems removed

1 to 2 stalks of celery with dark green leaves

1 cup fresh or frozen blueberries

2 peaches, pits removed

1 pear

½ avocado, pit and skin removed

4 dates, pits removed

2 tablespoons bee pollen (optional)

3 cups water

Cardio Workout Boost

▶ 2 cups purslane leaves

2 cups apple chunks

2 cups fresh or frozen cherries, pits removed

1 banana

2 sprigs basil

½ cup pomegranate juice

3 cups water

Endurance

▶ 2 cups beet greens

1 cup collard greens, stems removed

5 apricots, pits removed

5 dates, pits removed

½ cup pomegranate juice

½ avocado, pit and skin removed

3 cups water

Healthy Blood

▶ 2 cups kale, stems removed

1 cup parsley

2 cups grapes

5 fresh figs

Juice of 1 orange

1 sprig thyme

3 cups water

Body Balance

▶ 3 cups Swiss chard, stems removed

7 apricots, pits removed

5 dates, pits removed

Juice of 1 orange

2 cups water

Bone Builder

▶ 1 cup sunflower sprouts

1 cup dandelion greens

1 cup mustard greens

Juice of 3 large lemons

½ avocado, pit and skin removed

2 sprigs rosemary

2 cups water

½ cup alfalfa sprouts

3 tomatillos

Place sunflower sprouts, dandelion and mustard greens, lemon juice, avocado, rosemary, and water in a blender. Blend well. Pour into a bowl, add fresh sprouts and sliced tomatillos, and eat with a spoon.

Brain Boost

▶ 2 cups purslane leaves

1 cup fresh or frozen blueberries

2 cups fresh or frozen strawberries

Juice of ½ lemon

3 cups water

Brain Health

▶ 2 cups purslane leaves
1 cup spinach
2 cups fresh or frozen strawberries
1 banana
1 cup pomegranate juice
2 cups water

Creating Focus

▶ 2 cups Swiss chard, stems removed
2 cups fresh or frozen strawberries
1 cup unsulfured dried apricots that have been soaked
   in water for 1 hour
3 cups water

Memory Booster

▶ 3 cups spinach
2 sprigs rosemary
3 cups fresh or frozen blueberries
2 teaspoons chia seeds
3 cups water

Optimal Brain Function

▶ 4 cups purslane leaves

2 kiwis, peeled

2 cups fresh or frozen strawberries

3 cups water

Breath Remedy

▶ 2 cups wheatgrass

2 apples

2 mangos, pits and skin removed

Juice of 1 orange

Juice of 1 lemon

1 teaspoon cinnamon

3 cups water

Make-Out

▶ 2 cups parsley

2 apples

2 mangos, pits and skin removed

Juice of 1 lemon

3 cups kombucha

Halting Halitosis

▶ 1 cup wheatgrass

1 cup cilantro

2 cups fresh or frozen strawberries

1 apple

1 mango, pit and skin removed

Juice of 1 lemon

1 teaspoon cinnamon

3 cups water

Detox Starter Kit

▶ 1 cup wheatgrass

1 cup kale, stems removed

½ cup kelp (dried seaweed)

½ avocado, pit and skin removed

1-inch piece ginger root

2 cloves garlic

Juice of 1 lemon

3 cups water

Clean Blend

- 2 cups broccoli sprouts
- ½ cup cilantro
- 4 cups pineapple chunks
- ½ avocado, pit and skin removed
- 1-inch piece ginger root
- Juice of 1 grapefruit
- 3 cups water

Deep Detox

- 3 cups dandelion greens and flowers
- 4 cups pineapple chunks
- ½ avocado, pit and skin removed
- 1 teaspoon turmeric
- Juice of 1 lemon
- 3 cups water

The Ultimate Detox

- 2 cups collard greens, stems removed
- 1 cup cilantro
- ½ cup chives
- ½ avocado, pit and skin removed
- Juice of 1 lemon
- 3 cups water

Toxins Be Gone

▶ 2 cups stinging nettles

1 cup cilantro

3 stalks celery

Juice of 1 lemon

2 mangos, pits and skin removed

2 cups apple juice

Bright Eyes

▶ 2 cups green-leaf lettuce

1 cup horsetail

8 plums, pits removed

3 cups water

Healthy Eyes

▶ 3 cups spinach

5 cups papaya chunks

Juice of 1 orange

3 cups water

20/20 Vision

▶ 2 cups pumpkin leaves

1 cup purslane leaves

2 cups fresh or frozen strawberries

5 plums, pits removed

3 cups water

Eagle Eyes

▶ 2 cups beet greens

1 cup wheatgrass

3 cups fresh or frozen strawberries

1 mango, pit and skin removed

3 cups water

Healthy Eyes for Life

▶ 3 cups Swiss chard, stems removed

5 peaches, pits removed

Juice of 1 grapefruit

3 cups water

No More Gray Hair

▶ 1 cup wheatgrass

1 cup spinach

2 Hawaiian papayas, peeled, cut, and seeds removed

½ cup pomegranate juice

2 cups water

Heart Love

▶ 1 cup purslane leaves

1 cup green-leaf lettuce

2 cups apple chunks

2 cups black grapes

2 bananas

Juice of 1 lemon

3 cups water

Healthy Circulation

▶ 1 cup wheatgrass

1 cup pineapple chunks

2 cups fresh or frozen strawberries

1 medium cucumber, cut into chunks

½ cup cilantro

½ teaspoon nutmeg

2 cups water

Hormone Balance

▶ 2 cups spinach

1 cup beet greens

2 cups fresh or frozen blueberries

1 cup fresh or frozen cherries, pits removed

1 banana

3 cups water

Strong Immunity

▶ 1 cup wheatgrass

1 cup parsley

2 sprigs oregano

2 cups fresh or frozen blackberries

5 plums, pits removed

5 prunes, pits removed

Juice of 1 lemon

3 cups water (plus more if mixture is too thick)

Iron Boost

▶ 2 cups beet greens

1 cup watercress

3 mangos, pits and skin removed

3 dates, pits removed

3 cups water

Improving Hemoglobin

▶ 2 cups pumpkin leaves

1 cup parsley

1 apple

7 fresh figs

Juice of 1 orange

3 cups water

Love Your Joints

▶ 1 cup watercress

1 cup dandelion greens

2 cups fresh or frozen strawberries

1 cup pineapple chunks

2 sprigs basil

2 dates, pits removed

3 cups water

Kidney Support

▶ 2 cups butter lettuce

1 cup fresh or frozen raspberries

1 cup fresh or frozen cranberries

1 cup red grapes

1 cup young (Thai) coconut meat

Juice of 1 lime

3 cups water

Happy Kidney Function

▶ 2 cups parsley

5 cups cantaloupe chunks

½ lime, with peel

1 cup water

Lovely Legs

▶ 2 cups spinach

1 cup parsley

2 cups fresh or frozen cherries, pits removed

2 cups apricots, pits removed

3 cups water

Liver Cleanse

▶ 3 cups dandelion greens
2 apples
4 dates, pits removed
Juice of 2 lemons
3 cups water

Healthy Lungs

▶ 3 cups Swiss chard, stems removed
2 Hawaiian papayas, peeled, cut, and seeds removed
Juice of 1 lemon
3 cups water

Lung and Throat Opener

▶ 3 cups purslane leaves
2 cups fresh or frozen blackberries
1 mango, pit and skin removed
Juice of 1 lemon
3 cups water

Magnesium Blast

▶ 2 cups spinach
2 cups Swiss chard, stems removed
3 bananas
1 lime, with peel
3 cups water

Magnesium Champion

▶ 3 cups dock greens
7 prickly pears, peeled (wear gloves)
1 cup fresh or frozen blackberries
3 cups water

Magnesium Infusion

▶ 3 cups purslane leaves
3 cups fresh or frozen raspberries
1 cup fresh or frozen blueberries
3 cups water

Metabolism Boost

- 3 cups kale, stems removed
- 2 stalks celery
- 2 cups fresh or frozen raspberries
- 2 pears
- Juice of 1 lemon
- 1-inch piece ginger root
- 3 cups water

Women's Monthly Blend

- 2 cups Swiss chard, stems removed
- 1 cup dandelion greens
- 7 prickly pears, peeled (wear gloves)
- 1 mango, pit and skin removed
- 3 cups water

Potassium Blend

- 3 cups beet greens, stems removed
- 1 apple
- 2 bananas
- Juice of ½ lemon
- 3 cups water

Probiotic Berry Burst

▶   3 cups beet greens

2 mangos, pits and skin removed

1 cup fresh or frozen raspberries

3 cups kombucha

Probiotic Green Soup

▶   2 cups collard greens, stems removed

½ cup dill weed

1 cup unpasteurized fermented vegetables (carrots,
beets, ginger, daikon, cabbage, etc.)

½ avocado, pit and skin removed

1 red bell pepper, stem and seeds removed

2 cloves garlic

3 cups water

Raspberry Probiotic Drink

▶   3 cups kale, stems removed

1 cup fresh or frozen raspberries

2 mangos, pits and skin removed

3 cups kombucha

Sweet and Sour Green Soup

▶ 2 cups parsley

1 cup unpasteurized sauerkraut

½ avocado, pit and skin removed

1 red bell pepper, stem and seeds removed

2 cloves garlic

3 cups water

Beautiful Skin

▶ 2 cups kale, stems removed

1-inch piece fresh aloe vera leaf, with skin

7 apricots, pits removed

1 cup grapes

2 dates, pits removed

3 cups water

Glowing Face

▶ 1 cup plantain weed

1 cup fresh or frozen strawberries

1-inch piece fresh aloe vera leaf, with skin

½ cup young (Thai) coconut meat

1 cup water

Blend well. Eat with a spoon. Or apply to your face as a mask;
after 10 minutes gently wash off.

Good Night's Sleep

▶ 2 cups spinach

1 cup turnip greens

4 cups fresh, frozen, or dried tart cherries, pits removed

7 cherry tomatoes

1 banana

1 teaspoon raw honey (optional)

3 cups water

Sleepy-Time Smoothie

▶ 2 cups spinach

½ cup fennel greens

4 cups fresh, frozen, or dried tart cherries, pits removed

1 banana

1-inch piece ginger root

1 teaspoon raw honey (optional)

3 cups water

Sleep Like a Baby

▶ 2 cups spinach

1 cup watercress

4 cups fresh, frozen, or dried tart cherries, pits removed

5 guavas, any variety

Juice of 1 orange

1 teaspoon raw honey (optional)

3 cups water

Stress-Fighting Blend

▶ 3 cups lettuce, any variety

2 stalks celery

2 cups fresh or frozen blueberries

5 dates, pits removed

1-inch piece ginger root

Juice of 1 tangerine

3 cups water

A Calming Influence

▶ 2 cups Swiss chard, stems removed

2 cups pineapple chunks

2 mangos, pits and skin removed

3 dates, pits removed

3 cups water

Get-Happy Smoothie

- 1 cup dandelion greens
- 2 cups miner's lettuce
- 1 sprig mint or lemon balm
- 2 cups fresh or frozen strawberries
- 1 banana
- 3 cups water

Calming Nerves

- 3 cups spinach
- 2 star fruit
- 2 bananas
- 1 vanilla bean
- 3 cups water

Thyroid Support

- 2 cups Swiss chard, stems removed
- ½ cup kelp (dried seaweed)
- 2 cups pineapple chunks
- 1 large star fruit
- 1 mango, pit and skin removed
- 3 cups water

Calorie Burner

▶ 3 cups kale, stems removed

1 medium cucumber, cut into chunks

2 cups fresh or frozen strawberries

2 peaches, pits removed

Juice of 1 lemon

1 tablespoon young Douglas fir needles

3 cups water

Slender Blend

▶ 3 cups kale, stems removed

2 persimmons, seeds removed

1 cup fresh or frozen cranberries

6 dates, pits removed

3 cups water (plus more if mixture is too thick)

Slimming Blend

▶ 3 cups kale, stems removed

2 sprigs mint

4 cups watermelon chunks

1 cup fresh or frozen raspberries

½ banana

Juice of ½ lemon

1 cup water

Super Model

▶ 3 cups mizuna
1 apple
1 banana
1 cup fresh or frozen cranberries
3 cups water

Tropical Island Body

▶ 3 cups Swiss chard, stems removed
1 cup pineapple chunks
1 cup mango chunks
1 banana
2 cups water

Remedies & Relief

Bye-Bye Acne

► 2 cups dandelion greens

1 medium cucumber, cut into chunks

4 peaches, pits removed

3 dates, pits removed

2 cups water

A Natural ADHD Solution

► 2 cups beet greens

5 cups apricots, pits removed

3 cups water

Allergy Prevention

▶ 2 cups stinging nettles
1 cup spinach
5 kiwis, peeled
2 bananas
3 cups water

Allergic Reaction Relief

▶ 1 cup spinach
1 cup kale, stems removed
1 cup dried stinging nettles
5 kiwis, peeled
2 bananas
Juice of 1 lemon
1 teaspoon raw honey (optional)
3 cups water

Anti-Allergy Soup

▶ 2 cups stinging nettles
1 cup kale, stems removed
3 bell peppers, stems and seeds removed
1 avocado, pit and skin removed
Juice of 1 lemon
3 cups water

Anemia Prevention

▶ 1 cup grape leaves

5 stalks celery

3 cups fresh or frozen mulberries

1 banana

1 lemon with peel, seeds removed

3 cups water

Curing Anemia

▶ 1 cup borage greens

2 cups spinach

7 plums, pits removed

1 cup pomegranate juice

¼ cup kelp (dried seaweed)

3 cups water

Iron-Deficiency Recovery

▶ 2 cups Swiss chard, stems removed

1 cup kale, stems removed

3 peaches, pits removed

1 mango, pit and skin removed

3 cups water

Reversing Anemia

▶ 2 cups Swiss chard, stems removed

1 cup carrot-top greens

5 peaches, pits removed

1 cup grapes

3 cups water

Anti-Asthma Soup

▶ 2 cups Swiss chard, stems removed

2 sprigs basil

1 cup cremini mushrooms

2 tomatoes

½ avocado, pit and skin removed

Juice of 1 lemon

2 cloves garlic

3 cups water

Autoimmune Pain Buster

▶ 2 cups dock greens

4 cups fresh or frozen strawberries

1 banana

3 cups water

Autoimmune and Inflammation Defense

▶ 2 cups lamb's-quarters

1 cup kale, stems removed

1-inch piece fresh aloe vera leaf, with skin

5 large tomatoes

1 teaspoon turmeric

2 cups water

Mom's Best Friend, or Preventing Bedwetting

▶ 2 cups Swiss chard, stems removed

2 mangos, pits and skin removed

1 cup fresh or frozen cranberries

1 teaspoon raw honey (optional)

3 cups water

Remedy for Bladder Infections

▶ 1 cup plantain weed

1 cup spinach

3 cups fresh or frozen blueberries

2 cups fresh or frozen cranberries

3 cups water

IBS Relief

▶ 1 cup dandelion greens

1-inch piece fresh aloe vera leaf, with skin

1 mango, pit and skin removed

2 cups fresh or frozen blueberries

2 cups water

Note: If you feel discomfort from this smoothie, strain out all the fiber and drink only the juice.

Anti-Bronchitis Soup

▶ 2 cups spinach

3 bell peppers, stems and seeds removed

3 tomatoes

½ avocado, pit and skin removed

Juice of 3 lemons

2 sprigs oregano

3 cloves garlic

3 cups water

Bronchitis Relief

▶ 3 cups spinach

2 apples

2 mangos, pits and skin removed

Juice of 1 lemon

1 teaspoon cinnamon

3 cups water

Canker-Sore Eraser

▶ 2 cups Swiss chard, stems removed

1 cup cilantro

2 bananas

1 cup unsulfured dried apricots that have been
soaked in water for 1 hour

3 cups water

Carpal-Tunnel Relief

▶ 3 cups kale, stems removed

4 cups pineapple chunks

½ avocado, pit and skin removed

1 banana

3 cups water

A Typist's Best Friend

▶ 3 cups dandelion greens

4 cups pineapple chunks

2 mangos, pits and skin removed

1 banana

3 cups water

Celiac Symptom–Soothing Pudding

▶ 1 cup spinach

1 banana

1 mango, pit and skin removed

1 orange, peeled, sectioned, and seeds removed

1 lemon, peeled, sectioned, and seeds removed

1 sprig mint

1 teaspoon psyllium powder

1 cup water

Yield: 3 cups

A Gluten Gut Remedy

▶ 2 cups beet greens

1 cup fresh or frozen cranberries

5 dates

1 banana

1 orange, peeled, sectioned, and seeds removed

1 teaspoon chia seeds

1 cup water

Yield: 3 cups

Cholesterol Reducer

▶ 4 cups kale, stems removed

½ Mexican papaya, peeled, cut, and seeds removed

Juice of 1 grapefruit

2 cups water

Cholesterol-Lowering Soup

▶ 2 cups spinach

2 stalks celery

1 avocado, pit and skin removed

Juice of 1 lemon

3 cloves garlic

3 cups water

Cold-Sore Solution

▶ 2 cups beet greens
½ cup cilantro
5 cups apricots, pits removed
Juice of 1 grapefruit
2 cups water

Cough Cure

▶ 2 cups dandelion greens
1 cup spinach
3 mangos, pits and skin removed
Juice of 1 orange
Juice of 1 lemon
1 sprig oregano
3 cups water

Diabetes Prevention

▶ 2 cups dandelion greens

1 cup red-leaf lettuce

1 cup fresh or frozen cranberries

2 apples

1 cup young (Thai) coconut meat

3 cups water

Blood-Sugar Stabilizer

▶ 1 cup turnip greens (or mustard greens)

1 cup lamb's-quarters

2 large red bell peppers, stems and seeds removed

½ cup chopped green onions

Juice of 1 lemon

2 tablespoons chia seeds

1 tablespoon kelp (dried seaweed)

3 cups water

Low-Glycemic Purple Smoothie

▶ 1 cup romaine lettuce

1 cup grape leaves

1 cup fresh or frozen blueberries

1 cup fresh or frozen mulberries

1 tablespoon chia seeds

2 cups fresh or frozen blackberries

3 cups water

Reversing Diabetes

▶ 1 cup dandelion greens

2 cups beet greens

3 green apples

1 cup fresh or frozen cranberries

1 mango, pit and skin removed

2 teaspoons cinnamon

3 cups water

Diarrhea Remedy

▶ ½ cup raspberry leaves, fresh or dried

2 sprigs peppermint

2 scallions

2 very ripe bananas

1 cup dried blueberries

1 pear

1 cup apple juice

1 cup water

Eat slowly with a spoon.

Ear-Infection Fighter

▶ 2 cups romaine lettuce

2 bell peppers, stems and seeds removed

½ avocado, pit and skin removed

Juice of 2 lemons

2 sprigs basil

1 sprig rosemary

2 cloves garlic

3 cups water

Children's Ear-Infection Remedy

▶ 1 cup spinach
2 cups romaine lettuce
3 cups fresh or frozen blackberries
4 kiwis, peeled
1 mango, pit and skin removed
Juice of 1 orange
3 cups water

Preventing Edema

▶ 2 cups stinging nettles
1 cup spinach
1 cucumber, cut into chunks
2 bananas
3 cups water

Swelling Stopper

▶ 2 cups stinging nettles
1 cup young birch tree leaves
1 cucumber, cut into chunks
1 avocado, pit and skin removed
3 cups water

Swelling Pain Relief

▶ 2 cups stinging nettles

1 cup parsley

1 cucumber, cut into chunks

2 mangos, pits and skin removed

3 cups water

Tired-Eye Relief

▶ 2 cups spinach

½ cup cilantro

1 cup fresh or frozen mulberries

1 mango, pit and skin removed

2 cups fresh or frozen strawberries

3 cups water

Fever Reducer

▶ 1 cup purslane leaves

½ cup raspberry leaves, fresh or dried

Juice of 2 lemons

1 clove garlic

2 cups apple juice

2 cups water

Fibromyalgia Relief

▶ 1 cup wheatgrass

2 cups Swiss chard, stems removed

4 cups fresh or frozen blackberries

1 banana

3 cups water

Winter Flu Prevention

▶ 3 cups green-leaf lettuce

1 apple

1 cup unsulfured dried apricots that have been soaked
   in 2 cups water for 1 hour

1 cup apricot soaking water

2 cups water (plus more if mixture is too thick)

Gallstones Remedy

▶ 1 cup wheatgrass

2 cups dandelion greens

4 pears

1 cup fresh or frozen blackberries

1 cup grapes

Juice of 1 lemon

3 cups water

Gallstones-Be-Gone Soup

▶ 2 cups beet greens, stems removed

2 cucumbers, cut into chunks

½ avocado, pit and skin removed

Juice of 2 lemons

2 sprigs cilantro

3 cloves garlic

3 cups water

Gallstone Pain Aid

▶ 1 cup Swiss chard, stems removed

2 cups dandelion greens

4 cups papaya chunks

1 cup fresh or frozen raspberries

Juice of 1 lemon

3 cups water

Healing the Gums

▶ 2 cups sweet potato leaves

1 red bell pepper, stem and seeds removed

7 apricots, pits removed

1 tablespoon young Douglas fir needles

1-inch piece fresh aloe vera leaf, with skin

3 cups water

Hangover Cure

▶ 1 cup wheatgrass
½ cup mustard greens
3 bananas
Juice of 2 lemons
1 tablespoon raw honey (optional)
3 cups water

After-the-Party Helper

▶ 1 cup wheatgrass
9 prickly pears, peeled (wear gloves)
1 banana
Juice of 1 lemon
1 tablespoon raw honey (optional)
3 cups water

Heart Health

▶ 3 cups kale, stems removed
1 cup alfalfa sprouts
3 pears
5 prunes, pits removed
1 cup pomegranate juice
2 cups water

Heart Protection

▶ 1 cup buckwheat sprouts

1 cup turnip greens (or mustard greens)

1 cup arugula

1 red bell pepper, stem and seeds removed

3 large tomatoes

1 tablespoon chia seeds

Juice of 1 lemon

½ teaspoon turmeric

3 cups water

1 zucchini

Place all ingredients except zucchini in a blender. Blend well. Pour into a bowl, add fresh-grated zucchini, and eat with a spoon.

Heart-Healing Smoothie

▶ 2 cups miner's lettuce

1 cup purslane leaves

1 cup fresh or frozen cranberries

3 nectarines, pits removed

1 banana

3 cups water

Heartburn Remedy

▶ 3 cups kale, stems removed

1 cup fennel greens

4 cups cantaloupe chunks

½ banana

Juice of ½ lemon

1 cup water

Fast-Action Heartburn Relief

▶ 3 cups green-leaf lettuce

1 cup parsley

4 cups honeydew melon chunks

1 banana

Juice of ½ lemon

1 cup water

Heavy-Metal Neutralizer

▶ 2 cups bok choy greens

1 cup cilantro

2 mangos, pits and skin removed

1 apple

Juice of 1 lemon

3 cups water

Preventing Hemorrhoids

▶ 4 cups purslane leaves

2 kiwis, peeled

2 bananas

3 cups water

Natural Preparation H

▶ 3 cups stinging nettles

2 mangos, pits and skin removed

1 banana

1 tablespoon chia seeds

3 cups water

Preventing Hypertension

▶ 1 cup borage greens and flowers

3 stalks celery

5 guavas, with skin

1 cup fresh or frozen strawberries

Juice of 1 lemon

3 cups water

Blood-Pressure Regulator

▶ 1 cup watercress
1 cup green-leaf lettuce
1 stalk celery
5 large tomatoes
½ cup chopped green onions
½ avocado, pit and skin removed
Juice of 1 lemon
2 cups water

Fighting Infection

▶ 3 cups kale, stems removed
4 cups pineapple chunks
1 cup young (Thai) coconut meat
Juice of 1 lime
1-inch piece ginger root
3 cups water

Inflammation Cure

▶ 1 cup kale, stems removed

2 stalks celery

1 cup pineapple chunks

1 banana

4 kiwis, peeled

1 teaspoon psyllium powder

2 cups water

Yield: 3 cups

Anti-Inflammatory Blend

▶ 1 cup grape leaves

1 cup wheatgrass

3 cups fresh or frozen blackberries

Juice of 1 lemon

1-inch piece ginger root

3 cups water

Joint Relief

▶ 3 cups beet greens
1 bell pepper, stem and seeds removed
1-inch piece ginger root
Juice of 3 large lemons
½ avocado, pit and skin removed
2 cups water
½ cup fresh green peas
½ cup alfalfa sprouts

Place beet greens, bell pepper, ginger, lemon juice, avocado, and water in a blender. Blend well. Pour into a bowl, add green peas and alfalfa sprouts, and eat with a spoon.

Kidney Control

▶ 3 cups romaine lettuce
1 cup fresh or frozen cranberries
1 apple
4 dates, pits removed
3 cups water

(Anti-Kidney-)Stone Soup

▶ 1 cup dandelion greens

6 very ripe tomatoes

½ avocado, pit and skin removed

Juice of 2 lemons

2 sprigs basil

3 cloves garlic

3 cups water

Healing Menopausal Heat

▶ 2 cups kale, stems removed

4 sprigs sage

2 cups fresh or frozen strawberries

2 cups grapes

3 cups water

Reducing Hot Flashes

▶ 3 cups beet greens

2 cups fresh or frozen raspberries

2 cups fresh or frozen strawberries

1 tablespoon chia seeds

3 cups water

Easing Menopause

▶ 3 cups purslane leaves

4 prickly pears, peeled (wear gloves)

2 cups fresh or frozen strawberries

1 tablespoon chia seeds

3 cups water

Hot-Flash Remedy

▶ 2 cups wheatgrass

½ cup dried sage

3 cups grapes

1 cup fresh or frozen cranberries

1 banana

3 cups water

Migraine Relief

▶ 3 cups beet greens

2 cups fresh or frozen blackberries

1 banana

2 jalapeño peppers, stems and seeds removed

Juice of 1 lemon

3 cups water

No More Migraines

- ▶ 3 cups beet greens
- 1 cup fresh or frozen blackberries
- 1 banana
- 1-inch piece ginger root
- 3 cups water

Morning-Sickness Solution

- ▶ 2 cups romaine lettuce
- 2 sprigs mint
- 2 cups pineapple chunks
- 3 dates, pits removed
- 3 cups water

Morning Pregnancy Smoothie

- ▶ 2 cups Swiss chard, stems removed
- ½ cup peppermint
- 2 cups pineapple chunks
- 5 dates, pits removed
- 1-inch piece ginger root
- Juice of 1 lemon
- 3 cups water

Queasy Morning Cure

- ▶ 2 cups Swiss chard, stems removed
- ½ cup fennel greens
- 2 cups pineapple chunks
- Juice of 1 lemon
- 5 dates, pits removed
- 3 cups water

Natural Pain Reliever

- ▶ 1 cup red-leaf lettuce
- 3 sprigs thyme
- 1 cup fresh or frozen tart cherries, pits removed
- 1 cup fresh or frozen blueberries
- 1 banana
- 1-inch piece ginger root
- 3 cups water

PMS Cramp Cure

- ▶ 3 cups dock greens
- 10 fresh figs
- 1 banana
- 1-inch piece ginger root
- 3 cups water

Powering Through PMS

- 3 cups beet greens
- 2 cups fresh or frozen raspberries
- 1 cup fresh or frozen blackberries
- 1 banana
- 1 lime, with peel
- 3 cups water

Healthy Prostate

- 3 cups collard greens, stems removed
- 2 red bell peppers, stems and seeds removed
- 5 medium tomatoes
- ½ avocado, pit and skin removed
- Juice of 1 red grapefruit
- 1 clove garlic
- 2 cups water

Men's Anti-Cancer Soup

- 2 cups stinging nettles
  1 cup kale, stems removed
  3 bell peppers, stems and seeds removed
  3 tomatoes
  1 avocado, pit and skin removed
  Juice of 3 lemons
  3 cloves garlic
  3 cups water

Psoriasis Remedy

- 2 cups dandelion greens
  1-inch piece fresh aloe vera leaf, with skin
  1 mango, pit and skin removed
  2 cups fresh or frozen blueberries
  Juice of 1 lemon
  1 cup apple juice
  2 cups water

Sinus Blast

- 3 cups cilantro
  3 red bell peppers, stems and seeds removed
  1 jalapeño pepper, stem and seeds removed
  3 cups water

Tummy Settler

▶ 3 cups romaine lettuce

1 cup parsley

3 cups pineapple chunks

2 bananas

3 cups water

Natural Tums

▶ 2 cups bok choy greens

1 cup turnip greens

2 sprigs mint

5 nectarines, pits removed

1 cup young (Thai) coconut meat

1-inch piece ginger root

3 cups water

Acid Neutralizer

▶ 3 cups Swiss chard, stems removed

1 Hawaiian papaya, peeled, cut, and seeds removed

1 banana

Juice of 1 orange

2 cups water

Acid-Reflux Solution

▶ 3 cups romaine lettuce
1 cup fennel greens
4 cups papaya chunks
1 apple
Juice of ½ lemon
1 cup water

Preventing Varicose Veins

▶ 3 cups spinach
3 cups fresh or frozen cherries, pits removed
1 cup fresh or frozen blueberries
3 cups water

Getting Rid of Varicose Veins

▶ 2 cups spinach
1 cup parsley
2 cups fresh or frozen cherries, pits removed
2 cups pineapple chunks
3 cups water

Natural and Easy Weight Loss

▶ 2 cups parsley

1 cucumber, with peel

3 pears

Juice of 1 grapefruit

2 cups water

The Last Five Pounds

▶ 3 cups tatsoi

1 apple

2 cups grapes

¼ avocado, pit and skin removed

½-inch piece ginger root

Juice of ½ lemon

3 cups water

5 Success Stories

*Each new day is a blank page in the diary of your life.
The secret of success is in turning that diary into the
best story you possibly can.* —DOUGLAS PAGELS

Sleep Apnea Reversed, 60 Pounds Lost

My name is Ng Heng Ghee. In 2009, I was overweight and in poor health. I was 5 foot 9 inches tall, weighed 202 pounds, and had a body mass index of 29.9. The health report indicated that I should have an ideal weight of 155 pounds.

During that period, I started having dizzy spells and couldn't keep my balance. I became bedridden. I was desperate, as I didn't want to take medicine and wanted to heal completely. I went to seek help from several different Chinese physicians. I brewed traditional medicinal herbs to drink. I went to a clinic for traditional Chinese acupuncture, even the kind with electricity going into the needle. Nothing worked.

One day, I felt so bad that I took a taxi and proceeded to the emergency room at my local hospital. There, the doctor suspected that I could be having a stroke and immediately admitted me. They did many tests on me. I was told to walk in a straight line, which I could not do. A neurologist came to test my eyes, reflexes, and joint movement. I was given a CT scan. The results were inconclusive.

In the hospital, I slept a lot, and my reflexes improved so that I eventually could get out of bed. I stayed in the hospital for three days, and the doctors could not find anything wrong with me. They wanted to perform more tests, but I declined and asked to be discharged.

Call it fate or coincidence, I am not really sure which it was, but I happened to come upon the term "raw food" while doing some research on gardening. Somehow it led me to the Raw Family website, where I quickly ordered DVDs and books. While reading one book, I learned one man cured his sleep apnea by drinking green smoothies. I also suffered from sleep apnea, and the doctor who tested me in the clinic told me that I stopped breathing twenty-seven times in an hour! He gave me two options. One was to go for an operation, which would involve cutting open my throat to enlarge my airway. The success rate, he told me, was only 60 percent. The other option was to wear a sleep apnea device (CPAP) while I slept for the rest of my life. Before he could proceed with the operation, the doctor told me I would have to lose 20 pounds, because I had too much fat around my neck area.

"Why stop at 20 pounds?" I wondered. I decided to change my diet and lifestyle instead of going under the knife. So I started eating organic raw food. For the next week, I blended tomato, carrots, and beets in distilled water and drank it every day. To my amazement, my breathing became easier. My nostrils were no longer blocked. My energy improved tremendously. Within a month, I lost almost 20 pounds as well as 4 inches from around my waist. This was an incredible victory for me, as I had been putting on weight since 1997.

Excited, I watched all of the Raw Family videos, read all the books, and studied recipes. I immediately added green smoothies and dehydrated vegetables and fruits to my diet. My health got better and better and, within four months, I had lost a total of 55 pounds. I felt happy and never looked back. Today, I weigh 141 pounds. My body mass index is 20.9. My doctor was amazed, and he told me that whatever I was doing, I should continue doing it.

—*Heng Ghee*

Ulcerative Colitis Reversed

I will be forever grateful to green smoothies for saving my granddaughter Sara's life. I am convinced that, if I had not stumbled across Victoria's book, Sara would not be with us today.

At fourteen years old, my granddaughter had been suffering for months with rectal bleeding. She was going to the bathroom several times a day. Every time she went, there was bright red blood in her stool.

After several doctor visits, we still didn't have a diagnosis. Finally, doctors labeled her condition "ulcerative colitis" and put her in the hospital, where they administered high doses of steroids and glucose intravenously. Neither helped. The doctors wouldn't let Sara eat anything; their theory was, if there is no food, then she won't go. Later, we realized how wrong they were.

Meanwhile, a friend sent me an e-mail with an article about the benefits of greens, which I forwarded to my son and daughter-in-law immediately. A few days later, another e-mail came with a video of a young man describing the value of green smoothies. I forwarded that to my children. I became so inspired by this information that I decided to start making green smoothies for myself. After all, how could I ask my granddaughter to drink this "stuff" if Grandma didn't like it?

Initially, my son and daughter-in-law were skeptical, especially since the doctors warned Sara about fiber and fruit. Besides, it was almost impossible to deliver her green smoothies in the hospital.

But Sara's condition did not improve. She had dropped down to 79 pounds. She was constantly weak, and her blood count was very low. She was pale as the page you're currently reading. Finally, the doctors wanted to give her an injection of Remicade, which was known to cause many painful and serious side effects. Naturally, my son refused. Sara's doctor told my son and daughter-in-law there was nothing else to be done. "You might as well take the girl home," one doctor said. So my son and daughter-in-law did.

At home, they started giving Sara green smoothies. From day one the bleeding stopped. She still went several times a day, but what a joy—no blood! Sara continued drinking green smoothies twice a day with no sign of blood. She was quickly recovering. After about a month, an e-mail came from her parents with a picture of her first normal bowel movement in months! I am probably the only grandma in the world that was thrilled with a picture of real poop! Today, Sara is up to 102 pounds. She went back to school and is enjoying the life that a teenager should. She will be sixteen next March.

I will say till the day I die that green smoothies saved my granddaughter's life. I am so grateful for green smoothies!

—*Marlene Smith (Grandma)*

Healed Teacher Inspires
High-School Students

In February 2013, I came down with three undiagnosed symptoms—crusty morning eyes, pain in the upper knuckles of my hands, and continual body aches. I was surprised. I had always considered myself a healthy forty-three-year-old woman, one who exercises on a regular basis and eats a mainly raw diet without meat or dairy.

I decided to seek out information about natural remedies for my curious symptoms. During the summer vacation, I read two of Victoria's books, which inspired me to try green smoothies for breakfast. I started religiously drinking the green concoctions every morning. I was desperate to ease the multiple ailments I had been experiencing since February. Within a few weeks, my symptoms completely went away. I didn't hesitate to tell my doctors, who couldn't seem to help me, that green smoothies were the ultimate healer.

I continue to drink green smoothies today. If I'm traveling and don't drink them, I can tell. In October 2013, I drank my usual green smoothie and ran my best half-marathon time in the Baltimore Running Festival. However, two weeks later, when I traveled out of town to race in the Cape Cod Marathon, my digestive system was turned upside down from substituting a standard American breakfast for my normal green smoothie. As a result, I experienced major digestive issues on the course. If I ever run a marathon away from home again, I will take my blender with me.

Earlier this year, I applied for a grant, so I can prepare green smoothies with my students. I work at an inner-city high school in Baltimore, where my kids are surrounded by vending-machine food to fuel their young bodies. I want to teach them green-smoothie nutrition, so that they can improve their lives, just like I did.

—Linda Wilson

Chronic Pancreatitis Conquered by Chlorophyll

My name is Irina, and I am fifty-four years old. I live in Russia. Thanks to green smoothies, for the last three years I have been *living*, and not merely existing. Early in my life, I developed problems with my pancreas. Like many other young people, I didn't pay much attention to the pain, which only occurred from time to time. By 2005, however, I could no longer ignore it. Painful attacks followed every meal. The doctors, who hadn't yet learned how to treat the pancreas, simply tried to cover up the pain with cold packs, short-term fasting, and artificial enzymes.

I kept reading tons of literature, but to my great regret, information about chronic pancreatitis was very limited, and my condition worsened. In addition to pancreatitis I developed gastritis, cholecystitis, colitis, duodenitis, and a stomach ulcer. My energy dropped, because my body wasn't getting the necessary nutrition. At that time, my digestive system could only tolerate oatmeal and some cooked vegetables. I turned into a pale, sluggish, indifferent person, and I was increasingly visited by the idea of death as my salvation. Unable to witness my suffering, my daughter helped me search through bookstores, but we couldn't find any helpful books. But seek and ye shall find!

One day, I saw an advertisement for *12 Steps to Raw Foods*. I tried to go on raw food, but my doctor told me it wouldn't work for my condition. Unfortunately, in Russian medical school doctors don't learn enough about nutrition, and as a result they know too little about raw food and the importance of diet. Fortunately, I looked up Victoria's name on the Internet and bought her other book, *Green for Life*, which taught me about a woman who cured her pancreatic disease by drinking green smoothies. Sobbing, I thought that this was my chance!

In May 2011, I started drinking green smoothies. For the first four months, I drank them twice a day, in the morning on an empty stomach and in the evening after work, usually two to three cups of freshly blended green smoothie. I used lettuce, celery, and other leafy greens as well as bananas, apples, oranges, and water. If the bananas were not sweet, I added honey. Sometimes I added a pinch of sea salt. In the summer, I often used dandelion greens. In the winter, I grew sunflower and pea sprouts; I also grew oat grass and wheatgrass. Curiously, my cat, Alice, would sometimes come and eat my green grasses before I could get to them.

As soon as I started drinking my smoothies, I felt changes in my health. One time, after two weeks of drinking green smoothies, I awoke in the morning with the feeling that something was different. I noticed that I had absolutely no sweet cravings! For me, it was a huge change. The truth is I was always a big lover of sweets, in excessive amounts, since early childhood. Having no desire for sweets was a liberating experience for me.

As my pancreas continued to heal, my pain continued to recede. However, the detox symptoms made me nervous, sometimes even scared. Once, deep in my gut, I could feel itchy bumps moving along the path of the intestines. Now I understand that that was the worms coming out with the grass. They couldn't tolerate the alkaline environment created by the leafy greens. Similarly, a thick coating covered my tongue every morning, another sign of restorative cleansing. My eyes itched, and my eyelids swelled up, but all of that passed pretty quickly. Within a few days, I started experiencing bursts of energy. The gastric pains started to disappear, my mood brightened, and I wanted to live again, and more than ever.

I still drink green smoothies almost daily, but I also broadened my diet. I replaced white sugar with honey and fruit. I don't eat fried food, and I cut back significantly on my consumption of fat.

Both my daughters, who are twenty-seven and eighteen years old, drink green smoothies. My husband enjoys them too. He asks me to "please pour some fiber" for him. I printed out many copies of recipes for green smoothies, which I offer to friends whenever I have the chance. They listen to my story and agree that my solution is simple and inexpensive, but not everybody follows my advice. I hope they will remember about green smoothies if they need a health solution someday.

—*Irina Demidova*

Joint Pain and Anemia Reversed

I come from a family of arthritic, diabetic people. I started out taking naproxen to keep the pain at bay. At first I would only allow myself to take it when the pain was too intense to sleep. I progressed over the years to taking it every day, morning and night, exactly as written on the bottle.

Unbeknownst to me, I developed an ulcer. One day I went to work with an intense stomachache. I proceeded to work all day with the pain. Eight hours later, I stepped into my swimming pool to try to ease some of the tension in my gut. I couldn't handle the cold. The pain became worse. I began feeling exhausted. I returned to the house and decided to lay down with a warm rice pack on my tummy. I lay there for no longer than ten minutes when I felt an urge to vomit. Worried, I ran for the bathroom. My husband, who was in the bedroom, heard a thud. He found me lying on the bathroom floor, passed out.

I came around, dizzy and disoriented. I continued to pass out two more times as my husband tried to get me in the car. (I refused to go by ambulance.) We made the short trip to the emergency room. Less than a minute later I passed out again. When I came to, I was lying on a bed while nurses scrambled to take off my clothes and insert an intravenous line.

Doctors immediately started questioning me and my husband and found that I had gastrointestinal bleeding. I lost almost half my blood supply before they got the bleeding stopped. I spent the next several days in the hospital. I refused transfusions, because I knew I could rebuild my own blood. Slower, yes, but safer. I came home and followed the doctor's orders, but still didn't regain my energy. My hemoglobin would go up a couple points, then drop back down. After two months, it finally reached 12 grams per deciliter, the lower range of normal for women. I went back to work, but still felt exhausted. My hemoglobin dropped again. I battled exhaustion for the next two months, sleeping all the time I wasn't at work.

One day I saw an infomercial about a blender and green smoothies. Intuitively, I immediately ordered one online. Amazingly, after only a couple of days of drinking green smoothies, I felt more lively. Within two weeks, I was back in high-energy form, and I had dropped 10 pounds.

Today, my joints constantly feel healthy, and my blood sugar is stable. There is no doubt in my mind that the green smoothies saved me. Blending them allowed my body to absorb the nutrients I needed.

—*Kelly E.*

Allergies Gone, Along with 70 Pounds

I suffered from allergies my entire life. My symptoms included aching, exhaustion, insomnia, irritability, and intolerance for many common foods. Once I turned fifty, I started to put on weight—nearly 70 pounds. I needed to do something, or I would spend the rest of life sick and tired and lifeless.

I came across *Green for Life* and started to include a quart of green smoothies in my daily diet. At the same time, a new vegan restaurant opened in our area, which allowed me to eat healthy meals regularly with my friends. I didn't feel as if I were on a diet. I was simply enjoying my daily green smoothie and a veggie lunch or dinner—a mainly raw diet with green smoothies as the centerpiece of my daily menu.

The simple enjoyment of a quart a day of green smoothie completely transformed me. Within a year, I had lost 40 pounds, almost effortlessly, and almost all of my allergies had started to disappear. Since then, I've managed to get back to my weight from college, 125 pounds. I feel sixty-three years young. All my friends tell me I look "young and radiant." That's when I tell them about *Green for Life* or just give them a copy of this life-saving book.

—*Susan G.*

The Proof Is in the Smoothie

My family started drinking green smoothies every morning eight years ago. Like other green-smoothie advocates, we experienced many health benefits. Several months ago, however, I read a number of articles about the benefits of frozen wheatgrass juice, so I ordered some from a reputable company. My family and I started drinking the wheatgrass twice a day instead of our green smoothies. After a short period of time, I started experiencing tremors in my hand. I couldn't even sign my name legibly. The tremors continued for more than a month. I couldn't figure out what was wrong with me. My life became difficult; I couldn't work. One day it occurred to me that maybe it was because I wasn't getting all of the nutrients and fiber from my green smoothies. So I started drinking green smoothies again and—sure enough, within a day or two—my tremors ceased. I was back to normal, and I could sign my name. Don't ever give up your green smoothies!

—*D.J.*

Healthy Bowels for All

As a homeopath, I see a lot of patients who are on terrible diets. Although many of my suggestions fall on deaf ears, my patients suffering from constipation are always willing to listen. Talking about green smoothies is easy and quick. Everyone who tries them returns to my office saying how much healthier their bowels are. They also tell me that whenever they skip their regular green smoothie, they inevitably bind up again. That's right, a poor diet always results in poor bowel health. I am grateful to have a quick (and natural) fix available.

—*Madeleine Innocent*

Homeopath Prescribes Smoothies

I discovered green smoothies a few years ago. Since then, I have become a firm smoothie fan. I love experimenting with herbs and various flavors. I add them to my green smoothie, then ask my family or friends to guess its ingredients. Even the skeptics are often surprised at how good smoothies taste.

As a homeopath and colonic therapist, I of course recommend smoothies to all my clients, many of whom have discovered their enormous—and immediate—health benefits as well as the fun in blending them and how delicious they can be. I sometimes demonstrate how to make green smoothies at my clinic.

—*Frances B.*

Hypertension Healed with Green Smoothies

At sixty-two years old, I feel great. I am as full of energy as I was in my twenties. Here is my story. I grew up in a family of scientists in the Ukraine. My mother was a chemist and university teacher, my father a scientist in a technical field. As a child, I enjoyed the fact that my parents were able to explain to me everything I asked about. I was also fortunate to have brilliant teachers at school. So my grades were high, which earned me entrance into Kiev Medical University, which, at that time in the Ukraine, was about as likely as making it in Hollywood. To get ready for the exam, I studied with my mother every day at her lab in the department of forensic examination, where she would lock me in the training room so I could concentrate. I studied in there for hours, surrounded by cans and cans of medication.

While I was in school, I gave birth to my first daughter, so when I started working as a pediatrician, I was a young doctor and young mother. I remember feeling overwhelmed and disappointed, because even though I had the knowledge from medical school, the children were continuously suffering from multiple illnesses, including my own daughter. Pretty soon I realized that in reality I had become a postman who delivered prescriptions and permission slips. Frustrated with my own ineffectiveness, I started to learn alternative treatments and to prescribe them to volunteer patients. I began educating parents about acupressure, tempering the body, proper nutrition, herbal wraps, therapeutic baths, and other holistic methods. I also founded a small library for parents, where I conducted regular lectures about health. The topic was always the same: "Health for Your Children and You." The results were fast and positive, and the health statistic for my patients were the best.

Despite my enthusiasm, after a few months of my "double duties" I became very ill myself: constant headaches, back pain, and, later, hypertension. At that time, I read Paul Bragg's book about fasting and immediately applied it to my own health.

In 1990, my family moved to Israel, where I continued to spread the natural-health approach, for which I was punished many times by my bosses. In Israel, I became a vegetarian and stopped consuming wheat and dairy. I continued to practice short water fasts. When I added hiking to my routine, my blood pressure normalized.

In 2008, after we had moved to Canada, my health continued to decline. My hypertension continued. I often suffered from bronchitis, even pneumonia, and my blood pressure kept rising. Canadian doctors prescribed me some medicine and assured me that everything would be fine. But my health kept failing. At that time I intuitively felt that my health strategy had been missing something important. One day on the Internet, I heard a lecture by an Armenian health advocate, who mentioned Victoria's green smoothies. I ran to the local Russian store and bought all of her available books. First, I eagerly read a book per day, then started reading them slowly the second time. By the end of the week, I had become a raw-foodist and started drinking green smoothies. On October 12, 2012, I bought a new blender. It was expensive, but I believed that green smoothies and raw food were the missing pieces in my health plan.

At that time my husband and I delivered newspapers. We had to wake up at three o'clock every morning, regardless of the weather. Even though we tried to go to bed early, it was extremely tiring to get up every morning before dawn. We were always desperately sleepy. Soon after switching to a raw food diet, however, my husband and I were able to recover in five hours. At the same time, my blood pressure became perfect. As soon as my husband started drinking green smoothies, he decided to give up meat. And I lost the stubborn 10 pounds I had carried for twenty-six years.

Since then, I haven't been sick even once. Everyone continues to comment on my youthful appearance and shiny eyes. Naturally, I started trying to convert everyone around me to raw-foodism, but that was much harder than doing it myself. I noticed that it is easier for most people to drink green smoothies. All my children and my grandchildren enjoy them. Victoria's children's books are a big help in this endeavor. Occasionally, people laugh at me, but no power will ever move me from this rewarding journey.

—*Alona Ross*

Good-Bye Cigarettes

It first began in 2009 when my husband came home from a visit with friends in Perth, Western Australia. We had started liver cleansing, which included powdered greens in a probiotic formula. To me this seemed like enough greens already. His mention of a "green smoothie" made my gut wrench.

Nevertheless, two months later I got to visit our friends and was subjected to the green smoothie. I'm very particular about the taste and texture of food, so of course my brain was telling me that this was going to taste terrible, as most things good for you usually do. To my great surprise, this green smoothie tasted absolutely wonderful.

From that day on I have had a green smoothie every day, and these are the results. I lost 33 pounds in four months. I used to be a coffee-and-cigarette-for-breakfast type of person, and although I still have my coffee after my smoothie, I gave up cigarettes. I now only really crave healthy foods, and salads make me drool. Best of all, though, I noticed that as I became healthier, so did everything else around and about me. My thoughts, my actions all became healthy. When people ask me how I stay so slim and radiant, I always answer, "Green smoothies." If there is one thing you could do for your health, it is to add a green smoothie a day to it and embrace everything that comes with it.

—*Jodie Marshall*

Candida and Depression Corrected

I was introduced to green smoothies by accident when I noticed Victoria's book in the bookstore. It literally changed my life. At the time I was very depressed and desperate to get healthier. I did not know green smoothies would change my life so much for the better. By adding green smoothies to my daily diet, I was able to correct my candida infection and finally put an end to my constant craving and hunger pains. When I drink a smoothie in the morning, I don't get hungry until noon or two o'clock. And when I do get hungry, it's usually gradual. I stay energized the whole day, and my skin glows. My hair is shinier, and my eyesight is very clear. Though I am almost fifty, I look ten years younger, which I attribute to my green smoothies. My depression is gone, and I see the world in a completely different, more positive way. I share the green-smoothie miracle with as many people as I can.

—*Susan Nikseresht*

A Cholesterol Drop

I have always taken vitamins and supplements as far back as I can remember. A lot of this has to do with my military background (former U.S. Marine) and my regular gym attendance. It was not uncommon for me to spend between $100 and $200 a month on supplements. I remember one of the last supplements I took were phytonutrient supplements. Basically, a chemist would extract the good elements from plants and then heat-stamp them into a pill. I thought the idea was silly and thought to myself, "Why not just cut out the middleman and get the nutrients from the plant?" The only problem was that I hated fruits and vegetables with a passion. You would never see me eating an apple or an orange, and don't even think about putting anything green on my plate for dinner. So I continued with the supplements.

In 2012, I applied for a term life insurance policy. The insurance company wanted to get some lab work on me. I took their blood tests and was shocked by the results: cholesterol 285, HDL 54, LDL 201, triglycerides 147. That evening I happened to be watching late-night infomercials and was introduced to the concept of green smoothies and blending fruits and vegetables into a drink. I was intrigued. It seemed like a good way to kill two birds with one stone. I could get around my dislike for fruits and vegetables by drinking them, and I could cut my supplement cost by finally deriving nutrients straight from the source.

The next day I began doing an extensive online search for blenders capable of making green smoothies. I quickly eliminated just about all the ones featured on late-night television and settled on a good one, which arrived in January of 2013. Before rushing off to the grocery store to buy produce, I did a YouTube search on how to make green smoothies. One of the videos that popped up was "Green Smoothie Power" with Sergei Boutenko, so I watched that. I picked up a lot of good information from that video on what I could expect to happen physiologically, the importance of rotating greens, and one or two recipes.

The first morning I made a green smoothie, I was just pleased to have consumed something that was inherently good for me. One of the first things I noticed was how full I was. I went the whole day without eating. It wasn't until six in the evening that I sat down to have a meal. The next thing I noticed was that my blood-pressure diastolic number started to drop (I take my readings every morning). I also became less constipated, and my stool was lighter. By the end of the first week of consuming morning green smoothies, my craving for sugar started to wane. The first month on green smoothies I spiked them with stevia, but by week five the fruits and vegetables were sweet enough by themselves. The decrease in sugar intake in my diet tended to lift the "fog" around my brain and give me more clarity of thought.

Three months later, I decided to have a second set of labs done to see what changes were occurring at the cellular level. I was pleasantly surprised: cholesterol 250, HDL 47, LDL 180, and triglycerides 114. My improved lab tests motivated me to continue with the program. I added a few new recipes and a variety of greens (kale, collards, and Swiss chard, for instance). In September 2013, I had a third set of labs taken. The results: cholesterol 231, HDL 43, LDL 168, and triglycerides 98. Wow. A 54-point drop in total cholesterol, a 33-point drop in LDL, and a 49-point drop in triglycerides. Statins, it turns out, don't have anything on greens. The proof is in the numbers. I'm sold on green smoothies and have committed to making them a part of my personal lifestyle.

—*Matt Leatherwood Jr.*

Type 2 Diabetes Reversed

About ten years ago I was diagnosed with type 2 diabetes. Also, my blood pressure and my cholesterol levels were too high. From that moment on I had to take a series of pills, which I swallowed on a daily basis without worrying about side effects or alternative natural methods.

Every three months I went to the hospital to have my blood sugar checked. And every three months, the level gradually went up. It was not a good sign. Finally, in the spring of 2013 I was told I had to switch to a stronger medication. This time, I asked the nurse about possible side effects. She was very clear about this: my weight would increase considerably. I reacted on an impulse and said I was not going to take medicines that would cause weight increase, since this is something that has to be avoided especially by diabetic patients. I felt angry and needed some time to think about my situation. So I requested a new appointment in three months to reevaluate my health situation, and I left the hospital without the new medicines.

Having said these brave things to the nurse, I still felt very sad when I came home. To be honest, I had no clue where to start finding a solution for my health problems. I decided to contact Simone, my yoga teacher, who I knew was very health conscious. She was also a licensed foot reflex therapist, and I requested her help. After the foot massage therapy, Simone gave me a book about how to live longer by cutting back on quick carbs and replacing them with lots of fruits, vegetables, and whole foods. In general, no more bread and pasta and lots of vegetables instead.

Three months later, I went back to the hospital to have my blood levels checked. I will never forget the nurse's face as she read the results: my sugar level had gone down 1 full point! The nurse was very surprised and wanted to know everything about my new way of eating. I told her my story. In addition to the sugar level, my cholesterol and blood pressure were so much better that I no longer needed to take medication. I went home, happy and singing!

When Simone started to organize the Green Smoothie Workshop, there was no need to convince me to participate. Eating healthily had become my new lifestyle, and this was such a nice and tasteful addition to the numerous salads I was preparing for lunch every day. I really loved it! I purchased a high-speed blender and started preparing green smoothies every day. Now I take a green smoothie in the morning and at nighttime.

I had only one more final appointment at the hospital. The diabetic nurse checked my sugar level and again it had gone down another full point. No more medication was necessary at all, at last! I felt free! I have become addicted to my green smoothies. I even take my blender with me on vacations. As an additional gift I lost 18 pounds and feel energetic, full of life.

—*Ineke Marijnissen-van der Molen*

Severe Stomach Pain Reversed in Three Days

After giving birth to baby number five, I put on the extra weight and started feeling sick. I began having severe stomach pain all the time and did not know what was causing it. Over the next year, my gastroenterologist performed many blood tests, abdominal ultrasounds, and CT scans, an endoscopy, and even nuclear testing. He could not find anything wrong. At one point I became tired of going to the doctor, and I began to do some research on my own. This is when I discovered Victoria's books. I read all of them. Being so busy did not allow me to prepare meals for myself and something else for my family. The green smoothies were the answer. I could prepare a batch in the morning, store them in a glass container, and drink them throughout the day.

Within three days, I felt better. Impressed with my progress, my husband and oldest daughter started drinking green smoothies with me. Everyone began to ask me what I was doing to lose weight. I told them about the green smoothies. I no longer have anemia, constipation, or any of the other digestive problems that the doctor could not fix. I have much more energy when I drink a smoothie, and I crave vegetables more than any sweets or junk food.

—*A.R.*

Chronic Migraines Traded for Vibrant Health

I discovered green smoothies in the spring of 2009 when my health was seriously deteriorating and I decided that my doctors were only making things worse with prescription medicines. I was suffering with very bad acid reflux, bowel problems, including blood in my stools, and chronic migraines, which occurred at least twice a week. I'd also developed an increasing list of allergies. I even went for a cancer scan, because I was feeling so ill, and the passing of blood in my toilet terrified me. These symptoms did not appear overnight, but gradually crept up on me over several years. It was hard to believe that I used to be fit in my teens and twenties. I was an advanced student of the martial arts and considered myself knowledgeable about diet and nutrition.

As I hit my thirties (I'm now forty-five years old), however, my life took a different path, and I found myself running my own mail-order business, which kept me tied to my computer for the next decade. Gradually my weight rose from a healthy and lean 175 to a bloated 230 pounds. In retrospect, I can see that I developed an addiction to prescription painkillers for my migraines and bowel pain, and I became a regular social drinker and recreational drug user and smoker. Of course my choice of diet deteriorated into the lazy man's diet of processed food, takeout, sugars, and booze. I guess I was caught in a very typical male middle-age health crisis.

I finally started to confront my problems when one evening I experienced heart palpitations while socializing with friends. I didn't say anything to anybody, but for the next couple of nights I lay awake confronting my own mortality. I'd lost all faith in the medical profession. My doctors seemed not to care, and any medication I was prescribed seemed to make matters worse. As a last resort I turned to books and the Internet and started researching for myself, trusting my intuition. I soon came across the Raw Food online community, which impressed me, but was also a bit too radical for me at the time.

Then I stumbled across Victoria on YouTube giving a lecture about her family's journey from sickness to health via green smoothies. Her story in many ways mirrored my own. It also reminded me of my mother, who was suffering from a form of lupus and chronic asthma. She had been on medication for more than twenty years, and I feared she was close to the end of her life. Victoria truly inspired me, and the next morning I went out and purchased an inexpensive smoothie maker.

The idea of getting as much raw/live food into the body in a drink form was so obvious I was amazed that I didn't think of it myself. I've been a student of natural history and biology all my life (I'm now a wildlife photographer); I always knew that nature has all the answers and that my illnesses were largely to do with my filling my body with unnatural products and foods (poisons), which my body didn't know how to process.

My first week of green smoothies was basically about getting as many greens into my body as possible, lots of spinach, kale, celery, with a banana, a little lemon, and a slice of ginger root. I drank two quarts within an hour of waking up. I have to admit it took a few days to get over the initial taste, but within ten days I noticed a big improvement in my bowel functions. I also lost 10 pounds. I could really feel my body repairing itself, and within two to three weeks people started commenting positively on my appearance. I was now craving green smoothies and just good, natural nutrition. In addition I also started cultivating wheatgrass for juicing, something I highly recommend.

I threw myself into studying nutrition and started experimenting with wild foods. I also shifted from a diet of cooked food to an 80-percent raw-food diet. I also eliminated all the chemicals that I had taken for granted in my home environment. Five years later, all of my physical ailments have gone. No more meds. No booze. No other drugs. My weight is now a healthy 180 pounds, and my life is transformed in every way.

Because of my obvious physical and mental transformation, people started to ask what my secret was. Once I told them, most slowly started drinking green smoothies in addition to improving their overall nutrition. Like me, they experienced fantastic results. Best of all, my seventy-year-old mother broke away from her old habits and started taking a pint of green smoothie with me every morning. Her recovery has been astonishing. Her lupus has just about cleared up, as has her asthma. Although she still has to take a couple of her meds, she threw most of them into the trash bin. She's very active, the healthiest seventy-year-old woman I know. She preaches the virtues of her diet to anyone who'll listen.

Green smoothies and good, natural nutrition saved my life as well as my mother's. It is a big statement, but I stand by it. My journey has only just begun, but I'm looking forward to the rest of my life with vitality and freedom from disease. This fundamental knowledge should be taught in all schools; our society would be a better place if it regained its health and worked with nature instead of against it.

—*John Hodges*

Eczema and Asthma Gone

I start every day with a large green smoothie, and I would never replace it with any toast or cereals again. Here's why.

In my early twenties, my health condition deteriorated almost overnight. The eczema I had since my teens worsened. Showering was a nightmare. Lotions simply concealed the symptoms—not always effectively. I thought I would have to keep using them my entire life. In addition, I began my struggle with a year-round allergic rhinitis and asthma. I slept poorly and had difficulties studying, working part-time, and finishing everyday tasks.

Inhalers, nasal sprays, and lotions helped for some time, but this relief came to an end very fast. Now I had to deal with its side effects, such as nosebleeds, heart palpitations, and a deep, painful cough. Often I felt down, and my depression would provoke even more asthma attacks and skin inflammations.

At that time, I typically had one cooked meal per day, which consisted of vegetables, grains, pasta, and occasionally poultry and fish. The rest of the day I would eat chocolate, pastry, milk, cheese, bread, cereal, and pizza. Only when I started to have heartburn and digestion problems did I finally admit to myself that I needed to change my diet. First, I rejected processed food, along with my medications, which no longer worked. My husband and I switched to a vegan diet. This improved my health condition just a little, but my face, neck, and hands were still covered with painful inflammations, and my asthma attacks, while less intense, were still excruciating.

I knew there was still something wrong with the food I was eating. It became obvious to me that cooking destroys most nutrients. However, even then I did not realize that cooked food could be so closely associated with health. Eventually I learned more about eating raw and how various illnesses are healed with a raw-food diet. I was intrigued. I started looking for recipes online and couldn't believe how tasty raw meals looked, how alluring this food actually was. I recognized that all this time my body was craving raw nutrition. Once I had such a profound understanding, I couldn't stay the same and return to my old path.

As soon as I started drinking green smoothies, my eczema began to recede, and my breathing became much easier, regardless of the occasional bread and cereals in other meals. There was no more battling for air. My skin had also started to improve, regaining its elasticity. It no longer cracked, and there were no longer any red marks.

Before I started drinking green smoothies, I ate very little fruit and leafy greens in a raw form. After eating raw fruits, I would suffer from heartburn and bloating, which—I later learned—was generally caused by malnutrition and poor digestion. That has changed thanks to green smoothies. My digestion has improved a lot. Never in my life could I eat as many raw fruits and greens as I do now. This has led to the fact that, at the age of twenty-eight, I have so much more energy than I did when I was younger. Chocolate and pastry used to be my addictions. Now my cravings for them are gone. My mind is clear, and I feel calm.

After about three months, my husband and I switched to an almost 100-percent raw-food diet. We often drink the smoothie twice a day because it's so nourishing. It keeps us full for hours. After such a meal we don't feel tired or lethargic as we would usually feel after eating cooked food. Just the opposite. I feel as if the life energy is flowing freely through my body, healing it at the same time. While everyone around us has a cold or is fighting the flu, my husband and I always feel great! I took full responsibility for my health and then made a decision to bring it up to the highest possible level. Now I know that my life will be as I choose.

—*Karmen Bogatinovski*

Eczema Healed

I always considered myself a healthy person. I ate organically grown foods. I exercised. I slept fairly well. I felt life was good, and my health was great. Except for my hands. I had a small patch of eczema that started under one of my rings and slowly, over the course of a few years, engulfed both of my hands. It was excruciating! I had blisters that would itch, and I would scratch them until they bled; a throbbing, open wound was a welcome change from the unbearable itching. I couldn't sleep at night because the itching was too intense. A dermatologist gave me a prescription for a topical steroid. When I put it on, the itching stopped on my hands, but my arms broke out in the itchy blisters instead. I went to see a naturopathic doctor. He started me on homeopathic pills. These didn't help at all.

One day, a friend shared a green smoothie with me. As I started adding green smoothies into my diet, my hands cleared up. I didn't have to change anything else, I simply added green smoothies to my regular diet. This was the beginning of a journey to reclaim my health, which I hadn't realized I was losing. I kept the smoothies in my diet and eventually changed over to a mostly vegan diet, with the occasional piece of fish. Green smoothies saved me, and I didn't even know I needed them!

I realize now that the hand eczema was a warning sign, and had I not started drinking the smoothies, something much worse could have happened regarding my health. As a mother of three little ones, I simply can't afford any health problems. I'm so thankful for greens and the power they have to optimize my health. And what better way to get the nutrition I need than in a delicious, refreshing smoothie? Even my children love them!

—*Amber Wild*

Teaching Kids to Love Greens

Green smoothies are important not only for our health; they also offer a practical way to incorporate greens in the daily nutrition of every individual of any age.

Today, it has almost become ordinary and simple to mix and blend fruits and greens in a blender and to give the body as many good nutrients as possible and get the advantages of chlorophyll, liquid sun. Before 2004, when Victoria started the experiments with the liquefied greens, nobody thought about it. Though it is true that people consumed leafy greens, they usually only did so through raw salads. In January 2011, I had just finished reading Ann Wigmore's books about raw and living food, and I was wondering if anything new could possibly be found regarding raw food besides wheatgrass, almond milk, seed cheese, and sprouts. After watching Victoria's video, I realized that fruits and leafy greens were a great, natural combination and that green smoothies were a great contribution to the meaning of "living food."

As soon as I got my blender, I enjoyed experimenting with various tastes by combining fruits with different leafy greens from my own organic garden. In this way I consumed 70 percent more leafy greens than before I discovered smoothies.

My decision to start consuming smoothies did not come from any illness or health issue. I am in great physical condition, and I fortunately do not know what it means to feel sick. I never use medication. My family and I started to use green smoothies because we became convinced that leafy greens were even more important than we used to believe.

I did not notice a major difference in my physical health, but I did notice a big change in my thinking. I started to see things from a bigger, much broader perspective. For example, I see solutions that I have never considered before. I started to think about new, complex projects, visualizing them mentally. My creativity has also increased exponentially. Moreover, my sense of altruism increased considerably. I started to feel the need to create, initiate, and develop projects that could help people, especially children. Can green smoothies do that? Based on my own experiences, I can definitely say yes.

I believe that the best way to help change the world and the health of people is through teaching children to make the right food choices from the very beginning of their lives. Being a teacher and an organic gardener, I created a project in Romania called Copilul Verde ("The Green Kid"). I work with kids between the ages of four and six, teaching them what a healthy way of life means. During classes and workshops we make fresh juices, salads, and deserts. We decorate our dishes by carving funny animal figurines. We use the dehydrator, germinate seeds, and so on. I use the experiential learning techniques with fantastic results, and my little students are very happy. They go home after my class and ask their parents to put more leafy greens on their plates or they ask to blend fruits with greens.

I have so many nice ideas to convince kids to consume raw vegetables and greens that my classes have turned into seventy-five-minute shows that kids do not want to leave. Everything started from green smoothies. Now I see leafy greens differently. I now see the sun in them.

—*Luminita Alexandru*

Fatty Liver Reversed

I am a fighter. I started my wellness journey when my doctor told me that the fat levels in my liver were elevated. He basically accused me of being a drunk, even though I rarely consume alcohol. At home, I looked up "fatty liver," became scared, and started to wonder what I was doing wrong to cause this condition. I got various books on liver cleansing and started my own blog, which helped me learn more about wellness. I read that losing weight was important, particularly subcutaneous fat surrounding the organs. I am fifty-seven, so years of fat had accumulated. Don't get me wrong. I am not fat. I exercise and look okay for my age. However, this fatty liver business made me think *acutely* about longevity.

Adopting the diet change was easy enough, but I wasn't losing weight, especially weight around the middle. Then I discovered green smoothies and was immediately hooked. All that goodness in one simple drink with lemon, spinach, and fruits. I learned that lemon and spinach were particularly good for the liver. Three years into my new diet, I took another blood test, and it was all clear. My eye exam was also fabulous.

I still enjoy my daily green smoothie for breakfast. My diet is a lot simpler too. Everything I eat is almost always fresh, and I hardly ever eat any processed foods. I have lost 15 pounds—and counting.

—*Kaye Hillis*

No More Fear of Old Age

I had been searching for proof that there was a better way to age. As I watched people older than me getting sicker and sicker, I thought, "That's not the future I want for my family." I wanted to stay healthy, so I could enjoy our time together and not be slowed down by disease.

As I searched for a better way, I came across Victoria's website, which made so much sense I purchased *Green for Life* and read it all. My first smoothie was Strawberry Fields. I was so amazed at how tasty it was. How could something so simple and easy to make be so tasty and so healthy? I didn't expect to like green smoothies so quickly. But I have learned that it is the simple foods in nature, left in their natural state, that are always best for us. God wasn't wasting his time when he created all he did the way he did.

I love this new world of food. I have since learned about soaking, sprouting, fermenting, and dehydrating. I love creating smoothies, and I am excited about trying new things. I can't remember being excited about preparing food before. I am excited just typing about it. Even better, I no longer fear the future of my health, and I will be teaching my children so that they will be healthy too.

—*Lucille Rock*

Feeling Like Twenty at Fifty-One

My health has always been very important, because I'm aiming for a long and healthy life. I have found that green smoothies fit very well into this plan.

When I first discovered Victoria's book *Green for Life* and started with my green smoothies, I had already gone from vegan to raw vegan. At first, I didn't take my smoothies on a regular basis, because those blenders I bought only lasted for two months each and I wasn't able to buy the next one right away. I must have purchased five different blenders in those early days.

I suffered from stress, both because my youngest daughter was born severely premature and I divorced shortly thereafter. A year after my transition to raw food, I went to Victoria's lecture about green smoothies in Stockholm, Sweden. I not only learned a lot; I decided to incorporate green smoothies into my daily routine.

I had recently been told that I had an iron deficiency, probably from all the stress I had been through, in combination with breastfeeding plus the fact I had started jogging three days a week. My iron deficiency was so severe that the doctor rang the very next day and told me I should be picked up by an ambulance and get two bags of blood, but since I was so vital, it was enough that I took iron tablets. He also said that if he had been the one who was so low in iron, he would have been knocked out on the floor.

I never felt weak, mostly because of all the fruits and vegetables I ate, not to mention all the salad! However, I ran slower every time I jogged my round instead of running faster. My ankles and legs swelled up, and I got edema even though I did not eat any salt. After a week I went to the doctor and a blood test showed the deficiency.

Since I did not want to supplement, I added a lot more greens to my daily smoothie, mostly wild edible plants. My favorites were and still are nettles, thistles, and dandelions.

I got a hold of a very good blender, so I could have one to two quarts of my green smoothie every day. When I had a checkup later, my iron levels had gone up and I was not anemic anymore. It was great news.

The second piece of great news was from my dentist. For years, I had had the beginnings of a small hole in one of my molars. I also had had periodontal pockets for several years, and the depth had always been measured. After I had been drinking my green smoothies for a few months, I went to the dentist. Imagine my surprise when I learned that the hole was completely healed and all the tooth pockets gone!

When I had eaten raw food for a few years, I felt it was just too much nuts and fat, so I increased the amount to at least two quarts of green smoothie a day, sometimes more. Still, I ate vegetables for dinner. In the beginning, I was a little worried about my teeth because I ate so much fruit, but my dentist reassured me and told me that nothing I ate could nourish caries bacteria, and raw fresh fruits and leafy greens could not get caught up in the fine grid surrounding the teeth (as long as I only ate the way I did). I also had significantly whiter teeth, something I tried to get over ten years using whitening toothpaste without success. Earlier I almost got brown teeth because of all the tea I drank as a vegan and the nuts and fat I had when I was eating raw gourmet.

Ever since I was a teenager, I have had very dry skin. When it was at its worst, my thighs and upper arms felt like sandpaper. I had long tried to solve the problem and tried many different cures without success. I tried to eat more fat, more omega-3s, and more nuts and seeds and to drink more water, but nothing helped, and I had given up hope of ever getting good skin in a natural way. Previously I had used different moisturizing ointments, but after I became a raw-foodist I did not want to put anything on my skin that I could not eat. After nearly a week of green smoothies, I had, to my delight, baby-soft skin again.

Over the years, my eyebrows had become completely white and I am vain enough that it bothers me. After a few days with one to two quarts of green smoothie, I spotted the first dark hair in one eyebrow, and now the color is totally back in both.

But what surprised me the most was that my thigh muscle started to heal. Ever since I was a baby, I've had a pit in my right thigh muscle. It was 1 inch wide, 2 inches long and about ½ inch deep. After I started with green smoothies, the muscle slowly began to heal itself.

I have experienced so many health benefits just by changing my diet to raw food and green smoothies. Also my sight has improved, and I can now read without glasses. I am much happier now and feel a constant love in my heart. I still have my period; it comes as regularly as before, but I do not have the mood swings I had before.

My two youngest, who still live at home, also drink their green smoothies every day with a straw, and they just love them! It is good to know they're getting all the nutrients they need in the morning. The girls eat about 70–80 percent raw food and 20–30 percent gluten-free cooked vegan diet; in other words, they eat cooked vegan in school and raw food at home. On holidays, they eat mostly 100 percent raw.

Before I introduced raw food into our diet, the oldest was allergic to all red fruits and berries; she could not even eat yellow tomatoes or different colored bell peppers without getting rashes and sometimes even fever. The youngest had asthma and had several bad colds each winter. Often she did not even get well from her cough before she got sick again. She would cough for three to four months in a row. In just ten days the oldest became well from her food allergy, and the youngest became well from her asthma when they began to eat 80 percent raw food with green smoothies and cooked vegan without gluten.

I immediately notice the difference when they have not been drinking their smoothies in their mood and ability to sit still. If I'm late sometimes with making their smoothies, usually they ask if they're allowed to blend it themselves. They are six and eight years old.

It's amazing to see all the health benefits that come up. I am a fifty-one-year-old mother of six who feels like thirty and has the body of a twenty-year-old.

—*Mikaela Kayl*

Healing of Bad Injury Begun in Three Days

In June 2009, I tore my rotator cuff. In July while I was horseback riding on a street, my horse fell on me. Though I broke nothing, a severe infection developed in my leg. Eventually dead tissue developed above my knee that needed removal. My elbow, shoulder, back, hip, and leg, having hit cement, were painful and inflamed for months. Six months later, surgery was necessary to continue my active life and recover movement in my shoulder. I couldn't saddle my horse!

At this time I thought I was eating a well-balanced diet. I had cut out sugar and flour eight years earlier to lose weight. But by 2010 all I wanted to do was sit and knit. All my life I had been active, but now every time I tried to even do physical therapy, tendinitis would set in. I felt eighty years old instead of fifty-nine. When I asked my physical therapist why I couldn't seem to get rid of the pain, he said it was due to inflammation all over my body.

Around this time, a family member told me about green smoothies. While looking them up, I found Victoria's website, bought the book, and started drinking green smoothies. Maybe my dramatic improvement was due to the fact that my body needed fresh nutrients. All I can say is that after three days of drinking just two cups of green smoothie a day, my body was begging to go for a walk. It was such an unusual thought, I was actually shocked, but I followed the inclination.

I began feeling energetic and clear-headed. Of course, I started telling everyone, bought a blender, and have been drinking smoothies every day since. With this health improvement I continued reading about meatless diets. I started by taking all milk products out of my diet. Oh my gosh, what a difference that made in my allergies. That was the deciding factor for me. I had suffered severe allergies since I was eleven and my eyes would swell shut when I petted kittens. Then the seasonal allergies. This is an inflammatory response I had had all my life until I started to change my food.

My health problems before my accidents were six surgeries by the age of thirty-five, asthma, lung infections, colds, migraines, depression, skin conditions, arthritis, 55 excess pounds, prediabetes, and osteoporosis. I took three meds daily for seven months a year to manage the allergies.

I had bimonthly migraines that would last for five days at a time. Imitrex, acupuncture, and chiropractic treatments only managed them. My depression was so bad, I finally got meds for that too. I kept reading and was scared to become a vegan, but after seeing the dramatic improvement with green smoothies and removing milk I took the plunge.

I still sneeze a few times a day for maybe two weeks during the high-pollen seasons. My theory is that for fifty years I suffered the effects of a poor diet and have some damage that is not reversible. I have no asthma problems at all now, because I changed my diet and included green smoothies. Depression is a thing in the past, I rarely get a cold, my weight is perfect, and my migraines are few and manageable now. Arthritis is just barely noticeable once in a while, but not a concern. Diabetes is not a factor anymore. Skin conditions only flare up when some other injury taxes my body. And so far the osteoporosis is the same.

Now I am vegan, but have not gone all raw. A major portion of my food is raw and my health now is wonderful. I take no meds. Even when a rare condition raises its head, my body now has the power to fight it off and repair and heal itself. My blood stats are always great, with cholesterol down from 197 to 166, blood sugars within normal ranges, and blood pressure around 88/63. Mentally I am clear and happy. I will be eternally grateful to green smoothies, a delicious, easy way to improve health. Everyone can do this, even if it is the only thing they do. It has been my road to recovery.

—*Patt H.*

Notes

Author's Note

1. http://customers.hbci.com/~wenonah/new/howfindv.htm.

2. http://www.cdc.gov/chronicdisease/overview/index.htm.

3. "Study Shows 70 Percent of Americans Take Prescription Drugs," *CBS News,* June 20, 2013.

4. http://www.usatoday.com/story/news/nation/2013/10/17/obesity-rate -levels-off/2895759/.

5. Paul H. Keckley, et al., "The Hidden Costs of U.S. Health Care: Consumer Discretionary Health Care Spending," Deloitte Center for Health Solutions, Washington, DC, 2012, page 8.

Chapter 1: What We Learn in Childhood

1. Lise Eliot, *What's Going on in There? How the Brain and Mind Develop in the First Five Years of Life* (New York: Bantam, 1999).

2. Eckhard Hess, *Imprinting* (New York: Van Nostrand, 1973).

3. A. Varki, "A Chimpanzee Genome Project Is a Biomedical Imperative," *Genome Research* 10 (2000): 1065–70; S. E. Bassett, et al., "Protective Immune Response to Hepatitis C Virus in Chimpanzees Rechallenged Following Clearance of Primary Infection," *Hepatology* 33, no. 6 (June 2001): 1479–87.

4. Herbert M. Shelton, *Food Combining Made Easy* (Brighton, Canada: Willow Publishing, 1940).

Chapter 2: The Phenomenal Abundance of Nutrition in Greens

1. Dennis Goodman, *Magnificent Magnesium* (Garden City Park, NY: Square One, 2014).

2. http://www.webmd.com/heart-disease/guide/sudden-cardiac-death.

3. Stephanie E. Chiuve, et al., "Plasma and Dietary Magnesium and Risk of Sudden Cardiac Death in Women," *American Journal of Clinical Nutrition* 93, no. 2 (February 2011): 253–60.

4. http://www.mensjournal.com/health-fitness/health/magnesium-the -missing-mineral-20140117.

5. http://www.webmd.com/diabetes/news/20031223/magnesium-lowers -type-2-diabetes-risk.

6. K. Ziegler-Graham, et al., "Estimating the Prevalence of Limb Loss in the United States: 2005 to 2050," *Archives of Physical Medicine and Rehabilitation* 89, no. 3 (March 2008): 422–29.

7. http://ndep.nih.gov/am-i-at-risk/DiabetesIsPreventable.aspx.

8. http://ndb.nal.usda.gov/ndb/foods/show/2965?fg=Vegetables+and+Veg etable+Products&man=&lfacet=&count=&max=25&qlookup=Swiss+cha rd+&offset=&sort=&format=Abridged&reportfmt=other&rptfrm=&ndb no=&nutrient1=&nutrient2=&nutrient3=&subset=&totCount=&measur eby=&_action_show=Apply+Changes&Qv=3.4&Q5640=10.0&Q5641=1.0.

9. http://ndb.nal.usda.gov/ndb/foods/show/3214?man=&lfacet=&count =&max=&qlookup=&offset=&sort=&format=Abridged&reportfmt=ot her&rptfrm=&ndbno=&nutrient1=&nutrient2=&nutrient3=&subset= &totCount=&measureby=&_action_show=Apply+Changes&Qv=3.4&Q6 119=1.0&Q6120=1.0&Q6121=1.0&Q6122=1.0.

10. http://skipthepie.org/ethnic-foods/stinging-nettles-blanched-northern -plains-indians/.

11. http://www.newscientist.com/article/mg20126882.600-ancient-earth-was -a-barren-waterworld.html.

12. http://nutritiondata.self.com-foods-000138000000000000000-w.html.

13. Kate Rhéaume-Bleue, *Vitamin K2 and the Calcium Paradox: How a Little-Known Vitamin Could Save Your Life* (Toronto, Canada: Collins: 2013).

14. K. Nimptsch, et al., "Dietary Intake of Vitamin K and Risk of Prostate Cancer in the Heidelberg Cohort of the European Prospective Investigation into Cancer and Nutrition (EPIC-Heidelberg)," *American Journal of Clinical Nutrition* 87, no. 4 (April 2008): 985–92.

15. J. M. Conly, et al., "The Contribution of Vitamin K2 (Menaquinones) Produced by the Intestinal Microflora to Human Nutritional Requirements for Vitamin K," *American Journal of Gastroenterology* 89, no. 6 (June 1994): 915–23.

16. J. M. Seddon, et al., "Dietary Carotenoids, Vitamins A, C, and E, and Advanced Age-Related Macular Degeneration: Eye Disease Case—Control Study Group," *Journal of the American Medical Association* 272, no. 18 (November 9, 1994): 1413–20.

17. J. M. Stringham and B. R. Hammond, "Macular Pigment and Visual Performance Under Glare Conditions," *Ophthalmology and Visual Science* 85, no. 2 (February 2008): 82–88.

18. J. A. Mares-Perlman, et al., "Lutein and Zeaxanthin in the Diet and Serum and Their Relation to Age-Related Maculopathy in the Third National Health and Nutrition Examination Survey," *American Journal of Epidemiology* 153, no. 5 (March 1, 2001): 424–32.

19. http://www.mayoclinic.org/drugs-supplements/folate/safety/hrb-2005 9475.

20. http://www.cancer.org/research/cancerfactsstatistics/cancerfactsfigures 2013/index.

21. http://www.aicr.org/foods-that-fight-cancer/foodsthatfightcancer_leafy _vegetables.html.

22. S. Rokayya, et al., "Cabbage (Brassica oleracea L. var. capitata) Phytochemicals with Antioxidant and Anti-Inflammatory Potential," *Asian Pacific Journal of Cancer Prevention* 14, no. 11 (2013): 6657–62.

23. R. F. Baugh, et al., "Clinical Practice Guideline: Tonsillectomy in Children," *Otolaryngology—Head and Neck Surgery* (January 2011): 144 (1 Suppl): S1–30.

Chapter 3: Your A–Z Nutrient Prescription

1. http://www.garvan.org.au/news-events/news/how-coconut-oil-could-help -reduce-the-symptoms-of-type-2-diabetes.

Recipes Index

READERS SHARE THEIR SUCCESS STORIES

"I am down 13.6 pounds in under 2 weeks and almost arthritis- and fibromyalgia-pain-free. I'm singing your praises to everyone I can."
–Lorraine S.

"I want to thank you for making my life better after all these years of eating dessert for breakfast. I'm feeling much better, more positive, more clarity, focused, with more energy. After the very first shake I lost my cravings for sweets, and within 2 days my allergies began to clear up."
–Connie V.

"I did my measurements, and after just 10 days I lost 10 inches; 4 inches in my waist alone. I looked in the mirror and didn't see that gray fog around my face. I have energy! Headaches are gone! I have clear and alert concentration. I am healthy again! I am happy and feel younger, like a healthy 20-year-old. Thanks again, JJ. I will keep you posted. God bless you. "
–Divina A.

"I have lost 10 pounds. I lost 8 pounds the first week. I feel better than I've felt in a long time. My blood-sugar readings and blood-pressure readings are gradually coming down. My exercise is 3 to 5 days a week in water exercise at the local YMCA.

Thank you so much. I have fun saying I'm on the Virgin Diet. I'm 72. Thank you."
–Julia B.

"I lost 25 pounds in 2 weeks Thank you, thank you, thank you!"
–Samy B.

"I do want you to know that my husband and I are feeling so much better that I canceled my appointment with the gastro doctor. For that I want to say thank you. I haven't felt this good in a very long, long time."
–Karen & Bob G.

"My biggest issue was my diabetes and getting my blood sugar under control. For 3 years I tried every diet I could get my hands on. I wanted to treat my disease using diet and exercise rather than pharmaceuticals. Nothing was working. Some things worked for a while, and then after 2 weeks I was back where I started. I have been following JJ's program for a little over a month and things are just getting better. My blood sugar has leveled out. I have reduced my meals from 6 or 7 per day to 4. And my energy has increased."
–Marilyn E.

"After a lifetime of being hungry (I mean really stomach-growling hungry and overweight), I am now at peace. I am 53 years old and could hardly move because of joint pain. I had chronic irritable bowel syndrome, was ready for bed by 4 p.m. and was plagued by brain fog. Now I feel great, have so much energy, and I feel hopeful, no, *excited* about my future. Thank you for giving me back my life."
–Howard

"I've lost almost 10 pounds in 24 days with less effort than ever before. I haven't felt nearly as hungry on this diet as I have on *every other* diet I've tried. I'm not so hungry my stomach is sore, and I don't struggle getting to sleep at night because I sacrificed way too many calories in the day. What I'm trying to say is thank you so very much for putting this plan together."
–Tyler

"I wanted to lose the 7 pounds in 7 days. Well, I lost 11. I continued following the plan, and as of today have lost 34 pounds in 26 days! I am so excited, and for the first time in more than 10 years, I have no knee pain or back pain. Really, no pain of any kind. I am off all of the medications and have started exercising. That in itself was a miracle for me!"

–Belinda P.

"I am currently on Day 5 of your plan and have lost 5 pounds, feel great, and I am the best advertising you can imagine for your book."

–Gail R.

"I ate three full meals today and a snack. Now I got on the scale and discovered I lost 9 pounds in 9 days. I am amazed and feel fantastic. No bloating, intestinal issues or headaches like my "normal" day. My eczema is even clearing up. I had no idea I could feel like this."

–Angela S.

"For the longest time I accepted that my tummy excess was due to having children and gaining a combined 115 pounds from my pregnancies. But once I eliminated all of JJ's problem foods, for the first time since being a mom I had a flat tummy! All that time I was bloated and didn't know it!"

–Kirin Christianson

"You can imagine my surprise when I learned that a food I loved, and that I thought was keeping me skinny, was making me bloated, tired and irritable! Who knew? I love feeling wonderful, energetic and focused! Thank you, JJ! You transformed my life forever!"

–Lisa Sasevich